NURSE'S HANDBOOK OF
PATIENT
EDUCATION

NURSE'S HANDBOOK OF
PATIENT EDUCATION

Shirin Fali Pestonjee, RN, MS

SPRINGHOUSE CORPORATION
SPRINGHOUSE, PENNSYLVANIA

STAFF

VICE PRESIDENT
Matthew Cahill

CLINICAL DIRECTOR
Judith A. Schilling McCann, RN, MSN

ART DIRECTOR
John Hubbard

MANAGING EDITOR
David Moreau

CLINICAL PROJECT MANAGER
Beverly Ann Tscheschlog, RN

EDITOR
Margaret Eckman

COPY EDITORS
Brenna H. Mayer (manager), Priscilla DeWitt, Stacey Ann Follin, Shana Harrington, Jaime Stockslager, Pamela Wingrod

DESIGNERS
Arlene Putterman (associate art director), Susan Hopkins Rodzewich (project manager), Marianne Hughes (cover illustrator), Donna S. Morris, Joseph John Clark

TYPOGRAPHY
Diane Paluba (manager), Joyce Rossi Biletz, Valerie Molettiere

MANUFACTURING
Deborah Meiris (director), Patricia K. Dorshaw (manager), Otto Mezei (book production manager)

EDITORIAL ASSISTANTS
Beverly Lane, Marcia Mills, Liz Schaeffer

INDEXER
Kathleen Wasong

The clinical procedures described and recommended in this publication are based on research and consultation with nursing, medical, and legal authorities. To the best of our knowledge, these procedures reflect currently accepted practice; nevertheless, they can't be considered absolute and universal recommendations. For individual application, all recommendations must be considered in light of the patient's clinical condition and, before administration of new or infrequently used drugs, in light of the latest package-insert information. The author and the publisher disclaim responsibility for any adverse effects resulting directly or indirectly from the suggested procedures, from any undetected errors, or from the reader's misunderstanding of the text.

Printed in the United States of America. For more information, write Springhouse Corporation, 1111 Bethlehem Pike, P.O. Box 908, Springhouse, PA 19477-0908.

NHPE-   O
02 01 00 99   10 9 8 7 6 5 4 3 2 1

℞ A member of the Reed Elsevier plc group

**Library of Congress
Cataloging-in-Publication Data**
Pestonjee, Shirin Fali
Nurse's handbook of patient education / Shirin Fali Pestonjee
  p. cm. Includes index.
  1. Patient education Handbooks, manuals, etc.
  2. Nurse and patient Handbooks, manuals, etc.
  3. Health education Handbooks, manuals, etc.
  I. Title.
  [DNLM: 1. Nursing—methods Handbooks.
  2. Patient Education Handbooks. WY 49
  P476n 2000]
RT90.P47 2000
615.5'071—dc21
DNLM/DLC   99-36721
ISBN 1-58255-018-2   CIP

CONTENTS

PART III APPENDIX, SELECTED REFERENCES, AND INDEX

To Christopher,
a delightful guide to the important things in life;
Fali and Alice, my parents, for teaching me
about courage and resilience;
all the Pestonjees, Kotvals, and Aibaras
for the love that has always surrounded and supported me;
and the patients and nurses throughout my career
for the always fascinating, often heart-breaking,
and ultimately uplifting sharing of their hearts,
minds, and lives.

FOREWORD

Patient education is one of the most crucial aspects of nursing practice. When nurses engage patients during teachable moments, patients can be transformed. Symptoms subside, anxiety decreases, self-care improves, readmission rates decrease, quality of life increases, and knowledge of disease and treatment expands. Effective teaching and successful learning result in desirable outcomes.

Nurses' commitment to patient education is rooted in the patients' right to know what is happening to them, how to stay healthy, and how to regain their health. Patients need to be informed so that they can make appropriate and independent decisions.

Patients, family members, and friends rely on nurses for their educational needs. Nonetheless, opportunities for teaching and learning are finite in cost-conscious and time-limited health care institutions, homes, and community settings. Despite constraints, nurses find the time to teach patients when preparing for surgery, diagnostic procedures, and discharge, when friends or relatives are present, when explaining equipment, during treatments, when administering medications and helping with personal care, and during admission interviews. They teach at bedsides and in hallways, bathrooms, day rooms, triage areas, and classrooms.

Patients appreciate skills-oriented teaching, such as how to change dressings, self-administer medications, and perform postoperative exercises. Nurses also instruct individuals of different ages about lifestyle change, disease, illness and symptom management, preoperative and preprocedure preparation, laboratory values, and the necessity for follow-up care, safety needs, medications, and many other topics.

To promote successful teaching and learning, nurses take into account many learner characteristics. Preferred learning style, learning disorder, developmental level, ethnic group, sensory acuity, and mental status are some of the many factors that influence learning.

Other challenges of patient teaching remain. What is the knowledge level of patients at the beginning of the teaching-learning exchange? How do nurses know that patients have learned? Nurses rely on patients' verbal statements of facts; answers to questions; demonstrations of skills, procedures, and equipment use; questions about therapy and treatment; when to notify nurses and doctors about symptoms; evidence that medications have been self-administered as ordered; reports of adverse drug reactions; improvement in overall condition and laboratory study values; and increased mobility. A great challenge is to motivate patients to accept responsibility for their disease management.

Most nurses benefit from the structure of a formal teaching plan to focus on patients' immediate learning needs. Condensed, relevant guidelines, such as those included in this book, can help nurses who are short of time. Accurate, concise, relevant, and up-to-date information helps nurses to teach well and patients to learn efficiently.

Nurses' Handbook of Patient Education emphasizes successful teaching approaches for a wide variety of physical and psychiatric diseases. This book will enhance nurses' skills in patient education, a critical element of nursing practice and an essential part of improved patient outcomes.

Zane Robinson Wolf, PhD, RN, FAAN
Dean, School of Nursing
La Salle University, Pennsylvania

PREFACE

Over the past several years, nursing has diversified. Nurses practice in many areas besides the traditional hospital, clinic, office, and home settings. But all nurses — wherever they work — have one duty in common: They all have to teach.

Teaching is intrinsic to nursing, and it's each nurse's professional responsibility. But nurses already have several patient education books to choose from. So why this book? I'll give you several reasons.

First, *Nurse's Handbook of Patient Education* offers something most other patient education books don't. The typical patient education book focuses on either educational theory and process or the content to be taught for a given diagnosis. This book provides both. Part I is a succinct, easy-to-use framework for the teaching and learning process, and Parts II and III offer the reader an organized guide to the content the patient should learn.

Second, *Nurse's Handbook of Patient Education* recognizes that patients' literacy levels play a key role in their ability to learn. Functional reading and comprehension skills can't be assumed of any patient. This book shows nurses how to perform a general assessment of each patient's literacy level and how to choose appropriate teaching materials to ensure effective learning.

Third, *Nurse's Handbook of Patient Education* provides the reader with avenues for teaching patients from other cultures in ways that embrace and honor their values, beliefs, social structures, and dietary preferences.

Patient education often gets bumped to the bottom of the priority list by the more immediate physical needs of the patient and by the ever-growing demands on nurses' time. However, research studies consistently prove that patient education is the liberating key to better health and more judicious use of health care resources. I have written this book to remind nurses of the critical role of education in patient care and to help them accomplish it more fully as part of the priceless and blessed work they do.

Shirin Fali Pestonjee, RN, MS

ACKNOWLEDGMENTS

The popular and controversial African quotation "It takes a village to raise a child" is correct in my estimation; it just doesn't go far enough. I would add that it takes a village (at least) to maintain an adult, and I'm gratefully aware of what I owe to so many who have helped and encouraged me.

First, thanks to my family, both immediate and extended, and dear friends who have lightened the burden in many ways. Thanks also to the colleagues who have shared their patient education stories, their knowledge, their books, and their enthusiasm with me. I am grateful for the mission of Parkland Health & Hospital System and in debt to the patients and professionals there who prove, every day, that ingenuity, competence, and mercy are alive and well. Lastly, I want to thank Beverly Tscheschlog, my editor, for being so kind.

C hapter 1 provides a review of the basics, the patient's right to education, the nurse's legal responsibilities, keys to behavioral change, the difference between teaching and learning, the importance of communication, and the critical role of motivation in successful teaching and learning.

Chapter 2 covers the six basic stages of patient education: assessment, development of learning objectives, planning, implementation, evaluation, and documentation.

A s a nurse, you've seen firsthand the changing face of health care. Some of the changes have been small, some drastic. But one thing has become clear out of all the change and uncertainty: the increasing importance of patient education. Fueled by patient need, new legislative and accrediting mandates, and the recognition of the positive impact patient education has on health care costs and patient satisfaction, patient education has taken on a major role in health care.

If patient education must play such a major role, it needs closer examination. This chapter does just that, looking at the growing need for patient education, the main goal of education, the cornerstones of good teaching, and the importance of helping patients follow what they've been taught.

A GROWING NEED

Wherever you look in health care, you'll find mounting evidence of the growing need for patient education. You probably know firsthand the effects of diagnosis-related groups and managed care — earlier discharges, day surgeries for procedures that used to warrant longer hospital stays, more difficulty admitting borderline patients, the struggle to keep patients with limited home resources in the hospital for an extra day or two.

As a result, a great deal of care that once was done by health care professionals in the hospital is now done at home, often by patients themselves or their families, friends, or neighbors. And many of the procedures patients or their caregivers are performing — such as giving I.V. medications, flushing I.V. lines, and changing dressings — were once performed only by doctors or nurses.

Along with these tasks, patients and caregivers must also take on the subtler burden of medical decision making. Difficult decisions about what symptoms warrant a call to the doctor or a visit to the emergency department or whether a wound is healing properly are in their hands.

More home care means more teaching
If patients and their caregivers have to take responsibility for all this care, they need someone to teach them. Nurses and other health care professionals must take on the daunting task of teaching a great deal of material, sometimes in too little time, to patients who may not be willing, ready, or able to learn. This growing need for patient education has prompted major health care organizations to specifically address the role of patient education in health care. (See *Education: A patient's right.*)

A positive impact
Demanding as it is to provide so much patient education, it's encouraging to see the positive effects such teaching can have. Cost containment studies, for in-

stance, show that educating patients results in significant cost savings. Educated patients maintain better health and have fewer complications; as a result, they require fewer hospitalizations, emergency department visits, and clinic and doctor visits. For example, one 1997 study of patients with rheumatoid arthritis found that those who received patient education reported an increased ability to handle pain and fewer problems with the disease. Another study from the same year found that asthmatic adults who took part in a self-management program showed increased compliance with inhaled medication use. Patient surveys also show that patients are more satisfied if they feel they have been well taught.

Legal responsibility
Of course, patient education is important because it enhances patient health and satisfaction, but it's also your legal responsibility as a nurse. As expressed in a typical Nursing Practice Act, "The RN shall promote and participate in client education and counseling based on health needs." It doesn't happen often, but nurses have been taken to court over a failure or perceived failure to provide patient education.

THE MAIN GOAL

The growing importance of patient education is clear, but what is the main goal of such teaching? Is it just to make sure the patient learns the content and masters the skills he'll need?

These are necessary steps in teaching, and it's tempting to assume the job is done when the patient demonstrates that he understands the content and can perform the necessary procedures. However, those aren't the main goals of patient education. To reach the desired outcomes, patients must actually *change behaviors*.

You've probably experienced the difference between understanding a concept and changing behavior yourself. For example, you may want to lose 15 pounds or give up smoking. You understand what it takes. Knowing what to do doesn't automatically translate into the necessary changes in behavior — and you end up still carrying that extra weight or smoking those cigarettes.

Remember, when behaviors change, outcomes change.

Change isn't easy
Keeping in mind how hard it can be for you to change your behavior — even when you know exactly what you need to do — can help you recognize how difficult it can be for your patients. To help them reach the goal of changing their behavior, give them credit, praise, and encouragement for their efforts, and realize that bringing about changes in behavior is an ongoing process.

CORNERSTONES OF SUCCESSFUL TEACHING

Good patient education rests on certain cornerstones. Understanding these cornerstones can help you become a better teacher.

Recognize the difference between teaching and learning
It's easy to assume that if you've taught something, then surely the patient has learned it. Just think back to a complex and difficult class in school or college, though; did *you* learn everything just because it had been taught? Ideally, learning follows teaching — but not necessarily. (See *Teaching doesn't always equal learning*.) Keeping in mind the difference between teaching and learning, from assessment through documentation, can help you focus on what your patient has actually learned rather than what you've taught.

ROLE OF EVALUATION   If you can't assume that learning follows teaching, then you need to find a way to determine what the patient has learned. To do this, you'll need to shift your focus from teaching to evaluating learning.

Careful evaluation, using appropriate methods and tools such as return demonstration, discussion, and questioning, can help you determine what the patient has learned and what he hasn't grasped yet. A good documentation system can help you keep your evaluation of the patient's learning separate from your record of teaching methods and materials.

Establish and maintain the helping relationship

Old-fashioned as it may seem, the helping relationship — also called the nurse-patient relationship — is also crucial to patient education. Your patient won't be interested in learning from you if he doesn't feel that you care.

The following basic guidelines can help you establish and maintain a trusting nurse-patient relationship:

- *Show respect*: View and treat each patient as unique and worthwhile.
- *Build trust*: Act with integrity so that your patient can develop confidence in you and your abilities.
- *Demonstrate caring*: Show your interest in and concern for your patient.
- *Accept the patient*: Show your patient that it's safe to drop his defenses with you and that you accept him for what he is.
- *Be sincere*: Make sure your words and actions send the same message to the patient; this lets him know that you mean what you say.
- *Be a patient advocate*: Look out for your patient's rights and interests.

IMPORTANCE OF COMMUNICATION   Key to the nurse-patient relationship is clear communication. Good communication skills can help prevent misunderstandings from interfering with learning. Some of the most important skills include active listening, using open-ended questions, clarifying, validating, acknowledging and reassuring, and allowing silences.

Be an active listener

- Maintain eye contact to let the patient know you're interested and paying attention (some cultures consider eye contact inappropriate, but most patients are comfortable with it).
- Listen to your patient's spoken word with attention and concentration.
- Listen, too, for unspoken meanings as well as messages the patient may have trouble making clear to you.
- Observe the patient's nonverbal behavior. Is it consistent with what he's saying?
- Don't allow interruptions; frequent interruptions — such as speaking before the patient is finished, answering a call or pager, or letting others enter the room while the patient is speaking — will most likely result in the patient giving up his attempts to communicate with you.
- Respond in ways that encourage continued communication.

Use open-ended questions To encourage discussion, ask the patient open-ended questions. Questions that start with the words *what, when, where,* and *how* give the patient a chance to go into detail about an issue and can bring out information you might have missed if you asked a question that required a simple yes or no answer. Follow-up questions and comments — such as "Tell me more about that" — can bring out still more information. Keep in mind that questions beginning with *why* can seem threatening or judgmental. (See *Open-ended questions open up discussion.*)

Clarify Make sure you and your patient clearly understand each other. To help you do this, you can:
- *reflect* (repeat back to the patient all or part of his message)
- *paraphrase* (restate the patient's message in different words)
- *sequence* (review the events in a time sequence to make sure you understand what happened when)
- *summarize* (restate the important points and how they relate to each other).

Validate Check your interpretation of what the patient is telling you by stating what you think he's saying, both with his words and through his body language. Ask him if you've correctly interpreted his message.

Acknowledge and reassure Acknowledge feelings, both stated and implied, and reassure the patient that it's okay to express his feelings; the patient may be afraid to show feelings he thinks may make him seem weak or foolish. Letting him know that others also have such feelings and that his feelings are legitimate and worth discussing can give him much-needed reassurance.

Allow silence   Silence can give you and the patient time to think about what you've both said and what else you may need to talk about. It can also give you both a chance to choose the right words to talk about difficult topics and to deal with any feelings your discussion may have triggered.

Respect the patient's role
Patients arc becoming increasingly knowledgeable about their bodies. They have access to a wealth of information about health carc — on the Internet, in newspapers and magazines (many of which are specifically geared toward healthier living), and from television. And as patients learn more about how to stay healthy, they are taking a more active role in their own health care — a role that you need to recognize and respect. This growing involvement of patients in their own care is helping to change the approach of many health care professionals from the authoritarian "Do as I say" to the more cooperative "Here's why I recommend this."

In turn, your teaching and that of other health care professionals enhances the patient's role in his own treatment. Educating a patient about his condition, the benefits and risks of available treatments, alternative care options, and other health care information gives the patient the knowledge and understanding he needs to make appropriate decisions — and to be a respected part of his own health care team.

Don't make assumptions

Another cornerstone of patient education is recognizing that each patient is unique; you can't make assumptions about any of them. Your homeless patient may not be illiterate. Your wealthy, well-educated patient may not understand or comply with all your teaching. Your illiterate patient may prove quite capable of learning how to give himself insulin safely and accurately.

Avoiding assumptions also means that you need to recognize that people can change. The disinterested patient you saw last year may finally be ready to learn, and the patient who was doing so well before may have lost motivation and regressed.

Don't assume the patient has — or will use — all the resources needed to maintain his health. He may not have a refrigerator for storing his insulin. He may spend his money on cigarettes, even if that means he doesn't have enough left over to buy his medicine.

In all these cases, the antidote to assumption is to ask. When that helping relationship is in place, the patient trusts you enough to give you truthful answers. He knows you're not trying to judge or humiliate him but instead trying to give him the best care and teaching you can — care that fits his situation.

Understand yourself

Finally, you must know and understand yourself and recognize the need for continual self-evaluation and improvement. Recognizing and understanding your own views, values, perceptions, and expectations strengthens your ability to avoid assumptions about patients and helps keep you from imposing your biases on them. That, in turn, helps make you a better teacher.

Even so, recognizing your biases isn't easy. Thinking about the following questions can help you get started.

- *What are your health values?* You may believe that maintaining an appropriate weight, following a diet based on approved portions of the food pyramid, and keeping your teeth clean and intact are important health values. Your patient may not. By recognizing such differences, you can take the first step toward accepting the patient and developing a helping relationship.
- *What are your learning preferences?* You may be a visual learner who has to see it and read it (and highlight it) to learn it — but that's *your* preference. Your patient may learn best by hearing or doing, not seeing. Make sure your teaching repertoire includes methods and materials for reaching all types of learners.

- *How are your interpersonal and communication skills?* Are you so reticent that the patient thinks you're not interested in him? Do you continue on with the teaching plan even if your patient is fidgeting and looking out the window? Think about how your patient hears and perceives you. Look over the list of communications skills that appears earlier in this chapter, and make sure you're appropriately using the techniques suggested. Make changes as needed and see how your patients respond.
- *How are your teaching skills?* Ask for peer and learner evaluations. You may not always like what you're told, but reviewing and considering these evaluations carefully can help you make appropriate changes. Also, do objective evaluation tools show a correlation between what you think the patient has learned and what he actually has learned? If not, review all stages of teaching and learning; perhaps your skills need strengthening.
- *What are your professional motivations?* Are you sensitive about particular topics, such as having an abortion, refusing blood transfusions for children for religious reasons, or withholding a terminal diagnosis from a patient? Do your beliefs and feelings affect your teaching in these situations? Or can you remain accepting, nonjudgmental, and dispassionate and give your patients the professional care they need? If not, do you need to work in another situation?
- *What are your professional goals?* Do you believe that teaching is worth the time and effort it takes you to become proficient and to maintain your proficiency? Do you find teaching fulfilling, or would you be happier in a different role?

COMPLIANCE WITH TEACHING

By definition, *compliance* means that one must conform to another's wishes or rules. For the patients you're teaching, it means complying with what they've been taught. Even so, if the patient is truly in charge of making his own health care choices and decisions, then he shouldn't have to comply with any given health care professional's recommendations. He should be allowed to take those recommendations and do what he thinks is best for himself — even if that means ignoring medical advice.

This probably flies in the face of what you want for your patients. Of course you want each patient to make his own health care decisions, but you also want him to decide to use what you've taught him, to follow recommended treatments, to take his medicine as directed, to keep follow-up appointments — in short, to get well. If all patients "complied" with recommendations, more people would enjoy better health, many serious illnesses and disabilities could be prevented, and less overall time and money would be needed for health care. Not the least important, health care professionals would have the gratification of seeing positive results from their work.

Unfortunately, countless patients don't comply with health care recommendations, even if it's clear to their caregivers that they should. So how do you help your patients follow health care recommendations without forcing them to comply? What do you do when you know that the patient understands what he has to do, but he just won't do it?

When this happens, think through all the elements of patient education to see if you can put your finger on what may be keeping the patient from following health care recommendations.

- Make sure the helping relationship between you and your patient is in place.
- Make sure your biases aren't getting in the way.
- Reassess the patient's knowledge and skills. Go over material you thought the patient had learned; you may find that he has misunderstood or forgotten something important.
- Reassess the goals you and the patient are working toward, and think about who really chose the goals. Was it the patient — or you? If you chose them, work with the patient to establish goals he thinks are important, and make sure he understands the connection between changing his behavior and reaching the goal.
- Go over the patient's learning needs, style, and readiness. Would a different teaching method or setting make a difference? Is he emotionally ready to learn what you're teaching?
- Look again at what motivates this patient. Does he want to get well enough to enjoy his grandchildren? Or go back to work? Or does he lack the motivation to work toward better health? Sometimes the rewards of staying ill outweigh those of getting better.
- Reassess the effect the patient's financial situation may have on his ability to comply. Does he have to choose between buying food for the family and buying his antihypertensive drug? Should you consult social services?
- Review the patient's support network. Does he have the support he needs to comply? Do you need to get him help to set up a support system? Does he need a visiting nurse on an ongoing basis?
- Look over the specific behaviors the patient needs to change. Are they too complex for the patient? How can you break down the behaviors into manageable tasks?
- Think about how the patient views the cost of complying. Is that cost too great? For instance, does the patient think the benefit of undergoing treatment isn't worth suffering its adverse effects? Or is he unwilling to give up certain foods to lose weight?

Motivation

Despite your best efforts, some patients still won't follow health care recommendations. When this happens, you may need to turn from what may be interfering with learning and instead look at your patient's motivation.

Several theories address motivation — self-efficacy, coping, and attribution theory, to name a few. Understanding these theories may help you recognize what motivates a particular patient. This, in turn, can help you and the patient discover what you both can do to motivate him to improve his health.

For instance, attribution theory views people as being either internally or externally motivated. If your patient is internally motivated, he may balk at an outside authority telling him how to behave; he may respond better if you encourage *him* to take the lead in his recovery. If your patient is externally motivated, he may respond better to the directives of an external authority figure such as a doctor.

Throughout the patient education process, remember your goals — not only to help the patient learn what he needs to know, but also to motivate him to use what he's learned to change his behavior and improve his health.

A fter covering some of the basics of patient education, from the growing need for teaching to the difficult issue of patient compliance, it's time to look at the process of patient education. This process includes six basic stages: assessment, development of learning objectives, planning, implementation, evaluation, and documentation.

These stages commonly overlap; for instance, your evaluation may point to the need to go back and develop new learning objectives, and documentation takes place throughout the teaching process. Even so, each stage plays a distinct part in the overall process of patient education.

ASSESSMENT

Assessment of the patient's educational needs is the first step in the process. It gives you the basic information you need to create your teaching plan.

Why is an educational assessment important?

Assessment is an examination of the patient's condition — in this case, what the patient already knows, what he wants and needs to learn, what he's capable of learning, what factors might affect his learning, and what would be the best way to teach him.

Your assessment helps you find out what the patient already knows, which can save teaching time. It also lets you find out details about your patient that will allow you to tailor your teaching plan to his specific needs. Plus, it's an opportunity to get to know your patient, to develop a rapport with him, and to start building the helping relationship.

What should you assess?

Your educational assessment should focus on four major areas. Questions appropriate to each of these four areas can help you gather the information you need. (See *Sample assessment questions*.)

THE INDIVIDUAL First comes an overall assessment of the individual. The following are some specific areas you should assess.
- *Special needs*: Does the patient only speak a foreign language? Does he have a physical disability — poor vision, for example?
- *Support systems*: Does he have a loving, helpful family? Is he frail and alone? Is he homeless?
- *Health expectations*: Does he see practicing poor dental hygiene and getting dentures at a young age as normal? Does he view disability as a normal part of aging? Does he expect to remain healthy and vigorous even into his 70s and 80s?

SAMPLE ASSESSMENT QUESTIONS

These sample questions address the four major learning assessment areas and can be tailored to fit your patient's needs.

THE INDIVIDUAL
- What is an average day like for you?
- How has your average day changed since you've been sick?
- Who is most important in your life?
- What do you like to do in your spare time?
- Tell me about your family.
- Tell me about your work.
- What have you done in the past few years that you are proud of?
- How would you describe yourself?

LEARNING NEEDS
- What are your concerns about...?
- What do you feel you need to know to take care of yourself?
- What information do you need?
- What problems are you having with...?
- What do you know about your condition?
- What do you think caused you to become ill?
- What are you most interested in learning about?
- How will you manage your care at home?

LEARNING STYLES
- What time of day do you learn best?
- Do you like to read?
- What do you like to read?
- Would you prefer to read something first, or would you rather have me explain it to you?
- Do you remember something better if you read it, hear it, or try it?

LEARNING READINESS
- How do you feel about making the changes we've talked about so far?
- You don't seem interested in this information. Is there something else you'd like to talk about?
- Do you feel that what you're learning will help you to manage your condition?
- How do you think your condition will affect your day-to-day life?

- *Health values*: Does he eat fried foods, despite knowing their adverse effects on his health? Does he skip follow-up appointments to check changes in his blood pressure?
- *Cultural considerations*: Do his cultural values make it difficult for him to discuss intimate matters with a woman or accept her suggestions? How will his values affect his response to health care recommendations?
- *Financial considerations*: Does he have to live on a small, fixed income? Will he have trouble paying for his medications?
- *Personal factors*: What values drive the patient? Does he value taking responsibility for himself and others? Does he view acquiring of money and things as important? What are his interests? Maybe he likes playing Bingo or surfing the Internet. What's motivating him to seek health care? Being able to care for a grandchild? Getting back to work?

LEARNING NEEDS   Next, determine what the patient needs to learn. What does he already know about his condition? Does he have any misinformation you need to correct? What are his goals? Keep in mind that his goals may not be what you expect.

LEARNING STYLES   You'll also need to determine his preferred learning style. Does he learn best by reading (visual learner), hearing (auditory learner), or touching and doing (tactile learner)? What's his literacy level? How able is he to learn what he needs to know?

LEARNING READINESS   Finally, assess how ready he is to learn. Is his current health state interfering with his ability to learn? For instance, does just trying to breathe absorb all his energy, or is he too focused on pain to concentrate? Also, is he motivated to get well? Does he see himself as helpless in the face of his illness?

How you should perform your assessment?

You have several tools at your disposal to perform your assessment, including interviews and conversations with the patient and his family, observations, questionnaires and checklists, and conferences with other members of the health care team.

INTERVIEW THE PATIENT   Here's your chance to find out much of what you need to know directly from your patient. Does the patient tell you he's frightened and concerned? Do you notice that he's anxious, worried, or fearful? Does he say he's not interested in learning? What does he know about his condition? Has he already researched his condition and developed a plan of action? How has he coped with illness before?

INTERVIEW THE FAMILY   Interviews and conversations with the patient's family can fill in missing information, change your understanding of what you've heard from the patient, or affect your view of what the patient's home situation might be. For instance, does the wife's report of the family diet match the patient's? Does the family view the patient as a hypochondriac who should not be taken too seriously? Does the family tell you the patient has several drinks a day when the patient says he has only one? Is the spouse of a patient who has experienced a myocardial infarction willing to learn about a low-fat diet?

OBSERVE THE PATIENT AND FAMILY   During your interviews and conversations, observe the patient and family closely. Does the patient seem quieter and more depressed when his wife enters his room? Does the patient's wife reach to hold his hand when he has to have an I.V. started? Does a family member bring the patient ice cream and chocolate despite the patient's need to follow a low-fat diet? Do family members ask to be present during teaching? Do they participate?

USE CHECKLISTS AND QUESTIONNAIRES   Checklists and questionnaires can confirm information you've gathered from your interviews; give you further details about such personal information as diet, sleep habits, and levels of anxiety or depression; and help indicate the patient's literacy level and ability to write.

CONFER WITH OTHER HEALTH TEAM MEMBERS   Each health care team member sees different aspects of the patient. Conferring with others who care for the patient can give you — and them — a better picture, allowing you to develop a more complete assessment.

LEARNING OBJECTIVES

After the initial assessment, you and your patient will work together to develop learning objectives. This next step in the process helps to determine what the teaching plan will be like.

What are learning objectives?

Unlike goals, which are general and long-term, learning objectives are more specific, easily attainable, and short-term. For example, for a newly diagnosed diabetic patient, the overall learning goal may be to learn how to maintain blood glucose levels between 70 and 150 mg/dl at all times. Reaching such a goal may be overwhelming unless it's broken down into specific, short-term behavioral objectives that lead up to the overall goal. For this patient, an objective such as "After the lesson, the patient will be able to list five symptoms of hypoglycemia" is one step on the way to the overall goal of maintaining appropriate blood glucose levels.

What should you include in your learning objectives?

Learning objectives should include specific patient behaviors (such as listing five symptoms of hypoglycemia) that demonstrate what the patient has learned by a certain time (such as at the end of the lesson). More important, the objectives should include behaviors and indicate progress toward goals that you and the patient agree upon.

How do you write learning objectives?

Learning objectives should fit a five-part formula, clearly stating *who does what, how,* and *when.* (See *Writing effective learning objectives.*)

PLANNING

The next step in the process of patient education is developing your teaching plan. First, let's look at some key teaching guidelines as well as the different types of learners you're likely to encounter. Following these guidelines and recognizing the different ways people learn can help you develop better teaching plans.

Guidelines for effective teaching

These guidelines take into account certain shared characteristics of adult patients (for instance, that they want credit for their life experiences) as well as basic principles of teaching (for example, that conflicting information slows learning). They generally apply to the typical adult patient, although some also apply to any learner.

RECOGNIZE THE NEED FOR SELF-DIRECTION   Adults like to make their own decisions. Listen to what your patient believes he needs to learn and how he feels he would best learn it.

PROVIDE REALITY-BASED TEACHING   Adults want what they learn to have an immediate practical value, to meet a perceived need, and to fit their budget and time constraints. Remember, if the patient doesn't see any real value in what you're teaching, he won't pay attention.

GIVE CREDIT FOR LIFE EXPERIENCES   Adults want their individuality acknowledged and respected, so invite patients who have experience to share what they know.

ACKNOWLEDGE STRONG FEELINGS ABOUT LEARNING SITUATIONS   Many adults have strong feelings associated with learning — some good, some bad. Your patient may feel intimidated if he has to learn in a classroom-like setting, and he may not like authority figures such as teachers. On the other hand, he may have developed a lifelong love of learning. Observe your patient's reaction to different learning situations.

CORRECT MISTAKES SENSITIVELY   Adults can be sensitive to criticism, so correct mistakes they make gently. Point out what your patient understands or performs correctly first; then correct what he misunderstands or performs incorrectly.

RELATE NEW IDEAS TO CURRENT KNOWLEDGE   Learning and retention improve when the patient can connect what he's learning to something he already knows. Try to tie your teaching into your patient's hobbies, interests, and work.

RECOGNIZE THAT CONFLICTING INFORMATION SLOWS LEARNING   If your patient has seen another nurse perform a procedure one way and you're teaching him a different way, the conflicting information will slow his learning. You may be teaching him a slightly different way to follow sterile technique, for example, prompting him to say, "The other nurse didn't do it that way." You must then take the time to explain that sterile procedure (the key factor) isn't violated either way and give him a chance to reconcile the differences.

RECOGNIZE THAT LEARNING CAN CAUSE ANXIETY   The procedures you teach may seem routine to you, but to your patient, they're unusual and quite possibly frightening.

ALLOW ENOUGH TIME FOR LEARNING AND PRACTICE Another way to lessen your patient's anxiety about learning these new tasks is to make sure he has enough time to learn, practice, and ask questions.

ENCOURAGE ACTIVE PARTICIPATION The patient must be an active participant for learning to take place. Encourage discussion, questions, sharing of experiences, and (as appropriate) hands-on practice.

REINFORCE LEARNING Repeat key points many times to make sure your patient understands and remembers them. Expect questions.

PROVIDE A COMFORTABLE LEARNING ENVIRONMENT Make sure the learning environment is comfortable, both physically and emotionally. Give your patient support, keep your discussions confidential, earn your patient's trust, and make your patient feel special. Make sure he has everything he needs to learn better.

RECOGNIZE THE EFFECT OF STRESS Most adults lead stressful, hard-working lives. Recognizing this and acknowledging your patient's needs and individuality go a long way toward helping him learn.

Types of learners

Several systems categorize how people learn. The following two systems offer practical ways to categorize learning differences. Understanding these systems can help you devise effective teaching strategies that meet each type of learner's specific needs, which in turn can help you to develop better teaching plans.

GLOBAL AND LINEAR LEARNERS Global learners like to understand the big picture first and work their way down to the details. Linear learners want the details first and expect a coherent overall picture to emerge.

To understand the difference between these two types, think about how you would teach each one how to apply an elastic bandage. You would need to show the global learner a correct, completed example and explain the principles of applying elastic bandages before he would be ready to try it himself. You would have more success with the linear learner if you gave him step-by-step instructions and let him try them out; in the end, he would see that the finished product turned out right.

VISUAL, AUDITORY, AND TACTILE LEARNERS Visual learners learn best by reading, writing, and watching such visual media as videotapes and slides. Auditory learners need to hear information. Spoken explanations, lectures, and audiocassettes can help these learners, and they may remember information in pamphlets better if they hear it read aloud. Tactile learners must touch, manipulate, and perform a task to learn. Such a learner might remember more if he can touch and handle equipment; he may remember written information best by underlining or highlighting it.

Of course, each person uses a mix of learning styles but tends to rely more heavily on one style.

What is a teaching plan?
Now that we've laid some groundwork, it's time to look at the teaching plan itself. A teaching plan is a carefully organized, written presentation of what you and the patient agree he needs to learn, how you'll provide the instruction, and how you'll measure the results. A good teaching plan is your map. It shows the steps you and your patient need to follow to reach the learning objectives both of you have developed.

What should your teaching plan include?
Your teaching plan should include clear, concise teaching actions, including *what* will be taught, *when* teaching will occur, *where* teaching will take place, *who* will teach and learn, and *how* teaching will occur.

How do you develop a teaching plan?
Develop your teaching plan by focusing on each of the elements that make up the plan — the *what, when, where, who,* and *how* just mentioned.

PLAN WHAT TO TEACH Work with your patient to choose and prioritize learning objectives. Make sure you both agree that they address the patient's specific needs.

PLAN WHEN YOU WILL TEACH You'll need to consider several factors when planning teaching time.
- Take into account your patient's length of stay.
- Let the patient tell you what works best for him, and offer options. Does he prefer mornings, or does he have more energy in the evening? Does he like short sessions, or somewhat longer, more in-depth sessions?
- Assess how quickly the patient can absorb information. Ask him what kind of pace helps him learn best — slow and steady or more quickly.
- Ask the patient to tell you when he's tired so that you can continue later; watch for yawns, sighs, and indications of inattention.
- Keep teaching sessions relatively short — generally no more than 30 minutes and possibly as short as 5 minutes.
- You can't plan for these, but always be ready to grab those "golden teaching moments" when the patient is ready to learn — even when it means throwing your planned timetable out the window.

PLAN WHERE YOU WILL TEACH Consider comfort and privacy when you plan where to teach. For instance, if you need to have a long conversation with the patient, don't choose the uncomfortable chairs in the hall. If the patient is likely to cry or you have potentially embarrassing questions to ask, find an empty room with a door you can shut, or at least wait until the patient's roommate has left for a while. Make sure such distractions as noise, television, and the comings and goings of others don't interfere with your teaching sessions.

Also, consider other factors that might affect where you will teach, such as the size of a class or any special needs of your students. If you're teaching a class of 25 students, for example, don't teach in a room designed to hold 15. And don't teach your stroke rehabilitation class in a room that's a quarter mile from the parking lot.

PLAN WHO WILL TEACH AND WHO WILL LEARN As the patient's nurse, you're usually the primary coordinator of the patient's education, but other members of the health care team should also take part, including physical therapists, counselors, and other specialists. And don't overlook the role other patients can play. The American Cancer Society, for instance, has shown that having other patients visit can provide cancer patients with much-needed hope and motivation.

The person you're most likely to teach is the patient, but not always. You may also have to teach the patient's spouse or another caregiver, such as a friend or neighbor. If the patient can't care for himself at all or isn't capable of understanding what you teach — for instance, if the patient is a very young child — the caregiver may be your primary student.

PLAN HOW YOU WILL TEACH Carefully choose how you will teach based on what the patient or caregiver needs to learn and how he learns. Use your teaching strengths as much as possible, but don't get too comfortable with any one approach.

To meet each patient's needs, you'll need to have several teaching methods and types of materials at your disposal. Keep expanding your repertoire. But keep in mind that nothing can replace your interaction with the patient, no matter what methods and tools you employ.

Teaching methods You can choose from several teaching methods. As appropriate, use a mix of methods from the list below to meet your patient's needs:
- one-on-one sessions
- small-group discussions and support groups
- lectures
- demonstration and return demonstration
- role-playing
- games
- programmed instruction.

Teaching materials   Plan to use materials and teaching aids that fit your patient's learning needs. You can choose from several different types:

- pamphlets
- posters and flip charts
- videos and closed-circuit television
- computer-assisted instruction (diskettes, CDs, Internet)
- audiocassettes
- transparencies
- chalk or dry-erase boards
- models.

IMPLEMENTATION

You've made your assessment, set learning objectives, and created a teaching plan. Now it's time to implement the plan.

What is implementation, and why is it important?

Implementation is putting your teaching plan into action to reach the learning objectives you and your patient developed — in other words, it's the actual process of teaching. If you don't implement your plan effectively, your patient won't meet his learning objectives.

How should you implement your teaching plan?

To implement your teaching plan effectively you must tap into certain characteristics that are fundamental to good teaching. If you don't have all these characteristics, you'll need to work on developing them.

Implementing your plan well also calls for you to recognize the particular needs your patient has and to use the appropriate interventions. For instance, is your patient visually impaired? Is he homeless? Does he have poor reading skills? This last point is particularly important because more than 20% of adults read at or below the 5th grade level. If your patient falls in this group, you'll need to use teaching materials and methods geared to this reading level.

CHARACTERISTICS OF AN EFFECTIVE TEACHER   What makes teaching effective? Stop for a moment and think back to some of the teachers you've had — both good and bad. Consider the characteristics that got your attention, inspired you, made you want to do your best. These are the characteristics you'll want to develop as you teach patients:

- Know what you're teaching.
- Have passion for what you're teaching.
- Use effective communication skills.
- Develop and maintain the helping relationship.

- Show enthusiasm.
- Carefully manage the learning environment.
- Have a clear purpose, but allow flexibility.
- Use questions effectively.
- Apply behavior modification principles.
- Use emotions and senses.
- Understand the role of anxiety.
- Be sensitive.

SPECIAL NEEDS YOUR PATIENT MAY HAVE As mentioned earlier, your patient may have special needs that call for you to modify your interventions accordingly. If you don't take these needs into account, you won't be able to implement your plan effectively.

Visual impairment If your patient is visually impaired, don't assume he's also deaf. And don't assume he's helpless. Wait for the patient to ask for help before intervening. Also, remember that the patient can't see your expressions and body language, so he may misinterpret some comments.

Hearing impairment Many deaf patients can become easily frustrated and may have feelings of paranoia. Keeping the patient alerted to your presence and finding a workable communication system will help him feel included and respected.

Speech impairment Use tools that can help the patient communicate and decrease his frustration. Examples include letter and picture boards and a magic slate.

Homelessness A homeless patient faces many challenges. He'll have a hard time following a particular diet and finding liquids when he needs to take pills. He'll also have trouble trying to carry around necessary drugs, inhalers, syringes, crutches, and other equipment and keeping his medications and equipment from being stolen.

Lack of family involvement If the patient's family doesn't actively support him in his efforts to get well — for instance, if the family won't help a patient with heart disease follow his low-fat diet — the patient's job becomes doubly hard. Try talking with the patient and family members both separately and together to work toward creating a more supportive environment for the patient, and give your patient extra encouragement and positive reinforcement.

Low literacy skills and illiteracy Just because someone can't read well or at all doesn't mean he isn't intelligent. Because our culture highly values literacy, your patient may be reluctant to tell you that he can't read well or at all. You can't rely on his appearance or the number of years of school he has completed to judge his literacy level, but you still need to have some idea of his reading level.

Watch what your patient does. See if he makes a point of reading the newspaper; look around for evidence of other reading materials such as books or magazines. Does he read handouts you give him and ask logical questions that indicate comprehension of the material? Or does he glance at them and immediately put them down?

Listen carefully during your conversations. Does your patient routinely claim not to have glasses at the hospital and ask you to read handouts to him?

If your observations indicate that your patient can't read at all, modify your teaching plan to fit his needs. (See *Teaching the illiterate patient.*)

For the patient who can read only a little, choose reading materials that will give him every advantage. The following guidelines can help.

Content The written material you choose should:
- present essential information simply
- follow a basic how-to approach
- include only one or two key ideas in each paragraph
- include sensory information where appropriate (for example, the way a drug tastes or the feeling of warmth that injected dye can cause).

Style Try to choose written material that uses:
- a friendly, conversational style
- a simple question-and-answer format (when appropriate)
- simple, common, one- or two-syllable words (for example, "tell the doctor or nurse" rather than "notify the physician")
- consistent terminology (for instance, either *operation* or *surgery*, but not both)
- short, simple sentences
- the active voice (for instance, "take the tablet" rather than "the tablet should be taken").

Visual appeal Choose written materials that are printed in visually appealing, easy-to-read print. For example, slightly larger type is easier for most patients to read. Also, make sure everything isn't written in capital letters because that, too, can make the text more difficult to read. The text should use boldface or underlining or box information to emphasize important points, such as signs and symptoms that warrant a call to the doctor. In short, the written materials you choose should look easy to read, manageable, and inviting.

Pictures A patient with poor reading skills can gather a great deal of information from well-drawn pictures, so try to choose material that uses lots of illustrations. Simple line drawings, with only main items labeled, work best. Steer away from cartoon figures, too, because the patient may misunderstand them or view them as frivolous.

Look for pictures that show internal organs within recognizable outside body parts — for example, the lungs situated in the chest. Not all patients know the size and shape of internal organs. Also, choose drawings that show procedures being performed correctly and that show only the items the patient should use. That way, only the correct image remains in your patient's mind.

Inability to speak English If your patient can't speak English, remember that a kind face and a friendly smile work in all languages. If possible, use a professional interpreter; use family or friends to translate only as a last resort. (See "*But that's not what I said!*")

When working with an interpreter, follow these guidelines:
- Maintain eye contact with the patient — not the interpreter.
- Avoid medical jargon, slang, and idioms.
- Give the interpreter only two or three sentences at a time to translate, and give the patient time to respond.
- Maintain a good rapport with the interpreter.
- Allow extra time, usually more than twice as long you'd spend with a patient who speaks English.
- Don't put the interpreter in an awkward position by scolding or threatening the patient or by using swear words.

- Talk in a normal tone; don't raise your voice.
- Keep language phrase books and picture boards handy for communicating simple, neutral information such as "your lunch is here."

Cultural differences   Culture can have a profound effect on a patient's attitudes and beliefs about health care and can strongly influence his health care behavior. For instance, a female patient may not show up for follow-up care with a male doctor if her culture dictates that she should see only a female health care provider. If you regularly encounter patients from certain cultures, learn about those cultures, including a few key words of those languages. Most patients will be thrilled that you made the effort to learn a few words, even if your pronunciation isn't perfect.

When you're teaching, ask the patient to explain customs or dietary habits that you need to know about. Don't be afraid that you'll seem ignorant; the patient will probably be pleased that you're interested and that you care enough to ask. Try saying something like, "I don't know much about how the people of your culture cook food. Could you tell me about it?"

Wherever possible (as long as it's not contraindicated by doctor's orders or safety rules) and according to the patient's wishes, incorporate aspects of the patient's culture in your implementation. This may mean that you make time for daily prayer sessions, allow the patient to use special amulets or charms, or adapt care measures to fit the restrictions of holy days. Your efforts to accept the patient's customs and practices (and your apologies when you fail) will go a long way to reinforce the helping relationship.

Finally, keep your goal in mind. Your job is to help the patient learn how to handle his disorder, *not* to teach him that cultural beliefs (such as the belief that bad spirits cause illness) are not scientific and therefore wrong. Not only are such efforts usually unsuccessful but they also undermine the helping relationship.

Age differences   If your patient is a child, adolescent, or older adult, you'll need to gear your teaching to his age level. Often this means focusing your teaching on the caregiver.

EVALUATION

After you've started to implement your teaching plan, you'll need to evaluate how effective your implementation is.

What is evaluation and why should you evaluate?
Evaluation is the ongoing appraisal of the patient's learning progress during and after your teaching. It helps you determine how effectively you've implemented your teaching plan and what you may need to modify to help your patient reach his learning goals.

The most important reason for evaluation is to find out if your patient has learned what you set out to teach. But evaluation also reinforces correct behavior by giving the patient feedback on his progress.

What should you evaluate?
Of course, you should evaluate what your patient has learned and whether he has achieved his learning objectives. You should also evaluate every part of the teaching process. Did you and the patient develop specific enough learning objectives? Did the patient easily understand the pictures in the new material you used?

Next, you should evaluate your performance. Ask yourself these questions:
- Were you comfortable and at ease while teaching?
- Did you put the patient at ease?
- Did you make a comprehensive educational assessment?
- Did you help the patient set realistic learning objectives?
- Did you choose successful teaching methods and materials?
- Did you provide an emotionally and physically comfortable teaching environment?
- Did you teach at times when the patient was ready to learn?

- Did any new methods or materials you used work well? Why or why not?
- Did you choose appropriate evaluation techniques?
- Have you provided objective documentation of patient learning?

How do you evaluate?

Several tools can help you evaluate what your patient has learned. Some ways of evaluating include:
- watching return demonstrations to determine if the patient has learned the necessary psychomotor skills
- asking the patient to restate learned material to assess understanding
- asking questions and having conversations with the patient to pinpoint areas that need reinforcing or reteaching; careful attention to the patient's questions during these conversations may reveal misunderstandings or the need for more specific information
- giving written tests or questionnaires (as appropriate) before, during, and after teaching to measure cognitive learning
- conversing with the patient's family and other health care team members
- assessing physiologic parameters, such as weight and blood pressure
- assessing the patient's record of self-monitored blood glucose levels, blood pressure, and so on
- looking for evidence of behavior changes
- asking the patient to problem-solve in a hypothetical situation
- taping what the patient says or does (during a counseling session or during physical therapy) so that you and the patient can watch for patterns or specific behaviors.

To evaluate your own performance, you can ask respected colleagues to critique your teaching. You can also look over patient evaluations of your teaching. To critique your performance yourself, record or videotape your teaching sessions and look them over later.

Despite all the ways you can evaluate what your patient has learned and how well you've taught, evaluation can only go so far. It's not an exact science. To evaluate as accurately as possible, you'll need to work closely with your patient to find out what he has learned — and to determine what he still needs and wants to learn.

DOCUMENTATION

This part of patient education takes place throughout the teaching process. Documentation should start with the initial learning assessment and continue through your final evaluation.

You need to document patient education — both what you taught and what the patient learned — just as you do every other part of the nursing process.

What is documentation and why should you document?

The basic purpose of documentation is communication among health care team members. Good documentation helps maintain continuity of care and avoid duplication of teaching. It also serves as proof of the fulfillment of teaching requirements for institutional job descriptions and for regulatory and accrediting organizations such as the Joint Commission on Accreditation of Healthcare Organizations (JCAHO), provides a legal record of teaching and learning, and is mandatory for obtaining reimbursement from third-party payers.

What should you document?

A good documentation system should cover all aspects of patient education, including:
- any special needs the patient has
- the patient's learning needs, styles, and readiness
- the patient's current knowledge
- learning objectives and goals as determined by the patient and teacher
- information the nurse has taught
- teaching methods the nurse has employed
- objective reports of patient and family responses to teaching
- evaluating what the patient learned and how that learning was determined.

How do you document?

JCAHO offers these general guidelines to help you document effectively:
- Record the patient's name on every page of your documentation.
- Include the time and date on all entries.
- Sign each entry.
- Write in black or blue ink, for legal and reproduction purposes.
- Write legibly.
- Be accurate and truthful when discussing facts and events.
- Be objective. Don't show personal bias or let others influence what you write.
- Be specific.
- Be concise. Record information succinctly, without compromising accuracy.
- Be comprehensive. Include all pertinent information.
- Record events in chronological order.

Good documentation is a vital part of patient education. It not only serves as a legal record of what was taught and learned, it also acts as a means of communication among health care team members. And that helps improve the education process for all patients.

C hapters 3 through 15 focus on essential teaching topics that the nurse should review with a patient suffering from a major body system disorder: cardiovascular; respiratory; neurologic; immune and hematologic; gastrointestinal; renal and urologic; endocrine and metabolic; eye, ear, nose, and throat; musculoskeletal; integumentary; neoplastic; obstetric and gynecologic; and psychiatric.

The six primary areas of patient education are easy to remember, because their initial letters form an acronym for "MANTRA": **M**edications, **A**ctivity, **N**utrition, **T**reatments, **R**isk factors, and **A**ftercare. Usually associated with a mystical invocation or incantation, a mantra is also a word or motto that symbolizes a guide to action or a guiding principle. As you review teaching topics with your patients, then, let your "MANTRA" be your guide.

ANGINA PECTORIS

Defined as chest pain or pressure, angina occurs when the heart doesn't receive enough blood. The most common cause is coronary artery disease (see "Coronary artery disease," page 36), which results when atherosclerotic plaques constrict or block the arteries that carry blood to the heart.

Angina is a heaviness, tightness, or squeezing or burning pain in the chest that may radiate down the left arm, sometimes as far as the fourth and fifth fingers of the left hand. Less commonly, the pain radiates to the right shoulder and arm or up to the neck and jaw. It may be mistaken for gas pains, indigestion, or heartburn. The pain, which lasts for 2 to 15 minutes, is not usually severe. The patient may appear pale and sweaty, feel faint, and have heart palpitations.

TEACHING TOPICS

MEDICATIONS

- Nitrates (such as isosorbide and nitroglycerin) prevent or lessen anginal pain.
- Beta blockers (such as atenolol, labetalol, metoprolol, and propranolol) lower blood pressure, reduce the occurrence of anginal attacks, and control rapid heart rate.
- Calcium channel blockers (such as bepridil, diltiazem, nifedipine, and verapamil) lower blood pressure and reduce the frequency and severity of chest pain.
- Antiplatelets (such as aspirin) slow blood clotting.

ACTIVITY

- Regular aerobic exercise as tolerated; exercise should stop if angina occurs
- Avoidance of strenuous exercise

NUTRITION

- Small, nutritious meals (to avoid triggering anginal pain)
- Low-cholesterol, high-fiber diet
- Low-salt diet for hypertensive patient
- No gas-forming foods
- Rest after meals

Angina is considered stable when it has a predictable pattern of onset, duration, and severity and responds quickly (within 5 minutes) to rest and nitrates. Angina is considered unstable and a possible precursor to myocardial infarction (MI) if the onset of pain can't be predicted (for instance, if it occurs during rest or sleep) and doesn't readily respond to rest and nitrates. Variant (Prinzmetal's) angina is thought to result from spasms of the coronary artery and typically occurs during rest, usually early in the day.

POTENTIAL COMPLICATIONS
- MI
- Arrhythmias
- Sudden death

TREATMENTS
- Smoking cessation and avoiding second-hand smoke
- Planned exercise program
- Stress reduction and relaxation techniques
- Coronary artery bypass graft surgery, percutaneous transluminal angioplasty, stent placement, atherectomy, as appropriate in selected cases

RISK FACTORS
- Family history of cardiovascular disease
- Gender and age (men ages 30 to 55, postmenopausal women and women over age 50)
- Smoking
- High serum cholesterol level
- Other chronic diseases (such as hypertension, diabetes mellitus)
- Obesity
- Sedentary lifestyle
- Diet high in fat, cholesterol, calories, or salt
- Stress, hostility, and anger

AFTERCARE
- Tell the patient to:
  – avoid common pain triggers (large meals, major emotional stress, smoking, temperature extremes, high altitudes)
  – take medications as prescribed
  – have someone drive him to the emergency department if pain lasts more than 20 minutes without any relief or worsens.
- Tell the patient to seek help if the following occur:
  – chest pain that isn't relieved by rest and nitrates and lasts over 20 minutes
  – sweating or shortness of breath along with chest pain.

AORTIC ANEURYSM

An aneurysm is a bulge that develops at a weak spot in the wall of an artery or vein. Most arterial aneurysms occur in the aorta, probably because of the enormous pressure regularly exerted on the aorta during systole. Aortic aneurysms can be classified by *location* or *shape*. They can also be classified by *etiology*; causes include atherosclerosis (most common), congenital defects of the arterial wall, trauma, infections (such as syphilis), and hypertension.

Aortic aneurysms pose several risks. A thrombus that forms within the bulge can break loose and lodge in the brain or lungs, the aneurysm can cause pain or malfunction by pressing on nearby organs, or the aneurysm can rupture, in many cases with fatal results.

TEACHING TOPICS

MEDICATIONS

- Antihypertensives (such as clonidine) lower blood pressure by vasodilation, decreasing the risk of rupture.
- Beta blockers (such as atenolol and propranolol) also lower blood pressure.

ACTIVITY

- No strenuous exercise, heavy lifting, and activities such a snow shoveling
- Alternating periods of activity with rest to prevent overexertion

NUTRITION

- Low-salt, low-fat diet
- No caffeine (because of its vasoconstrictive effects)

Most aortic aneurysms don't cause direct signs or symptoms; they may be found on X-ray or when examining the patient for another problem. Signs and symptoms that do occur may result from pressure on nearby structures — a thoracic aneurysm, for instance, may cause breathing difficulty, coughing, blood in the sputum, hoarseness, or difficulty swallowing, and an abdominal aneurysm may cause abdominal, groin, side, or back pain and a pulsing epigastric mass.

POTENTIAL COMPLICATIONS
- Pressure on and decreased blood supply to organs or limbs
- Dissection
- Emboli
- Myocardial infarction
- Rupture (in many cases fatal)

TREATMENTS
- Achieving and maintaining appropriate weight
- Aortic aneurysm repair if symptoms occur, if the aneurysm increases in size, or if the size on initial assessment is greater than 4.5 cm (greater than 6 cm in patients who are poor surgical risks)

RISK FACTORS
- Atherosclerosis
- Gender and age (men ages 50 to 70)
- Congenital defects (such as Marfan syndrome)
- Hypertension
- Trauma
- Infections (such as syphilis)

AFTERCARE
- Tell the patient to avoid aspirin (because of its anticoagulant effect).
- If blood supply to any part is diminished, provide extra skin care precautions.
- Tell the patient to seek help if the following occur:
  – severe headache
  – sudden, severe pain in chest, back, abdomen, or groin
  – fainting
  – confusion
  – unusual restlessness or anxiety.

ARRHYTHMIAS

Arrhythmias are abnormal heart rhythms. Several types exist, ranging in severity from mild to life threatening, but all affect how much blood the heart pumps out. They can be classified by *origin* (atrial, atrioventricular junctional, or ventricular [the most dangerous]), *rate* (tachycardia or bradycardia), or *conduction malfunction* (heart blocks).

Arrhythmias can result from several causes, including insufficient blood supply to meet the heart's needs (which can also result in angina, myocardial infarction, or heart failure), electrolyte imbalances (particularly potassium), lactic acidosis, and drug toxicity.

TEACHING TOPICS

MEDICATIONS

- Antiarrhythmics help keep heart rhythm normal and regular.
- Digitalis glycosides increase the force of ventricular contractions and slow heart rate.
- Beta blockers lower blood pressure, reduce the occurrence of anginal attacks, and control rapid heart rate.
- Calcium channel blockers lower blood pressure and reduce the frequency and severity of chest pain.

ACTIVITY

- No overexertion; exertion should stop if symptoms occur
- Regular aerobic exercise
- No driving if arrhythmia causes periodic dizziness or faintness

NUTRITION

- Potassium-rich diet (helps prevent arrhythmias from low potassium levels)

Signs and symptoms depend on where the arrhythmia originates, heart rate, and conduction pattern and generally indicate the strength of cardiac output. If cardiac output is strong, the patient may have no symptoms. Weaker output may cause the patient to tire easily and have palpitations, chest pain, dizziness and faintness, shortness of breath, sweating, anxiety or confusion, and peripheral edema. Ventricular tachycardia and fibrillation can result in a loss of consciousness, seizures, and sudden death.

POTENTIAL COMPLICATIONS
- Heart failure
- Asystole
- Emboli
- Cardiac arrest

TREATMENTS
- Pacemaker insertion
- Automatic internal cardiac defibrillator insertion
- Carotid sinus massage
- Valsalva's maneuver
- Oxygen administration
- Smoking cessation
- Stress reduction and relaxation techniques

RISK FACTORS
- Myocardial ischemia
- Toxic levels of some antiarrhythmics, beta blockers, and angiotensin-converting enzyme inhibitors
- Hyperthyroidism or hypothyroidism
- Congenital heart disease
- Vagal stimulation
- Electrolyte imbalance (potassium, sodium, calcium)
- Inflammatory heart disease (rheumatic fever, pericarditis, endocarditis)
- Electric shock

AFTERCARE
- Teach the patient with atrial fibrillation how to check carotid, not radial, pulse.
- Suggest that family members take a cardiopulmonary resuscitation course.
- Tell the patient to seek help if the following occur:
  – fast, hard heartbeat
  – irregular heartbeat
  – heart rate five or more beats slower than preset pacemaker rate (if applicable)
  – chest pain
  – shortness of breath
  – dizziness
  – fainting.

CORONARY ARTERY DISEASE

Coronary artery disease (CAD), sometimes also called ischemic heart disease, remains the leading cause of death in this country. It underlies many conditions and may remain undetected until a patient seeks treatment for another condition, such as angina, myocardial infarction (MI), or heart failure.

CAD is a narrowing of the blood vessels that supply the heart with blood. This narrowing of the arteries diminishes blood flow to the heart. As a result, the heart receives insufficient oxygen and nutrients and responds with pain (angina). If oxygen deprivation is severe and prolonged, the affected heart muscle dies (MI).

CAD usually results from atherosclerosis. In this disorder, fatty plaques of cholesterol and lipids build up over time on the inside walls of the arteries, narrow-

TEACHING TOPICS

MEDICATIONS

- Antilipemics reduce the level of certain protein and fat combinations in the blood.
- Antiplatelets slow blood clotting.
- Beta blockers lower blood pressure, reduce the occurrence of anginal attacks, and control rapid heart rate.
- Calcium channel blockers lower blood pressure and reduce the frequency and severity of chest pain.
- Nitrates prevent or lessen anginal pain.

ACTIVITY

- Regular aerobic exercise as tolerated; exercise should stop if angina occurs
- No isometric activities (such as straining during a bowel movement, heavy lifting, pushing or pulling)

NUTRITION

- Low-fat, low-sodium diet with limited caffeine intake to lower blood pressure; patient must check food labels for fat and sodium content
- Preferred cooking methods: broiling, microwaving, grilling, and roasting
- Supervised, safe dieting for overweight patient
- Limited alcohol intake (up to two drinks per day, with the doctor's approval)

ing and, if unchecked, eventually occluding the arteries. CAD develops over years and appears to start in childhood, most likely because of the high-fat, high-calorie diet and sedentary lifestyle that is typical in the United States.

POTENTIAL COMPLICATIONS
- Angina
- MI
- Cerebral vascular accident
- Heart failure

TREATMENTS
- Smoking cessation
- Stress reduction and relaxation techniques
- Estrogen replacement in postmenopausal women
- Coronary artery bypass graft surgery, percutaneous transluminal angioplasty, stent placement, atherectomy, as appropriate

RISK FACTORS
- Family history of cardiovascular disease
- Gender and age (men ages 30 to 55, postmenopausal women and women over age 50)
- Smoking
- High serum cholesterol level
- Other chronic diseases (such as hypertension, diabetes mellitus)
- Obesity
- Sedentary lifestyle
- Diet high in fat, cholesterol, calories, or salt
- Stress, hostility, and anger

AFTERCARE
- Tell the patient to stop activity and take nitrates if angina occurs.
- Tell the patient to seek help if the following occur:
  – chest pain (crushing, tightness, or aching)
  – pain or discomfort in the neck, jaw, throat, shoulders, back, or arms
  – nausea, severe indigestion, or heartburn
  – a fast or irregular heartbeat
  – difficulty breathing, particularly at rest
  – sweating, dizziness, or feelings of weakness.

DEEP VEIN THROMBOSIS

Deep vein thrombosis (DVT) is a condition in which thrombi form in the deep, large veins of the leg, usually in the calf or popliteal area. Thrombus formation is thought to result from slowed blood flow, a quicker clotting time, and damage to the inside lining of the vein wall (Virchow's triad).

Some patients have few, if any symptoms. Others may have a slight fever, skin discoloration, pain, tenderness, warmth, and swelling of the leg. Patients at risk for DVT require screening, close monitoring, and preventive treatment because of the risk of a thrombus breaking free and lodging in the lungs or brain — a leading cause of death in the United States. Ultrasonography and impedance

TEACHING TOPICS

MEDICATIONS

- Anticoagulants (such as warfarin or low-molecular-weight heparin) prevent further clot formation.

ACTIVITY

- Monitored exercise program
- No standing for long periods
- No sitting with legs crossed or dangling; legs should be elevated

NUTRITION

- Adequate hydration
- Healthy diet based on recommended portions from the food pyramid

plethysmography are used for detection and monitoring. Prevention methods include early ambulation when possible, antiembolism stockings, intermittent pneumatic leg compression, and administration of low-molecular-weight heparin, low-dose heparin, or both, as indicated by the patient's level of risk.

POTENTIAL COMPLICATIONS
- Pulmonary embolism
- Cerebrovascular accident
- Recurrent thrombus formation
- Chronic venous insufficiency
- Venous stasis ulcers

TREATMENTS
- Antiembolism stockings
- No garments that bind legs (knee-high or thigh-high stockings)
- Smoking cessation
- Achieving and maintaining appropriate weight
- Surgical implantation of filtering device into the vena cava to trap emboli before they reach the lungs, if anticoagulants and thrombolytics are contraindicated

RISK FACTORS
- Prolonged bed rest; hospitalized patients, particularly after surgery, are at increased risk for DVT
- Obesity
- Varicose veins
- Pregnancy and childbirth
- Use of oral contraceptives

AFTERCARE
- Tell the patient:
  –to practice foot care for stasis ulcers, including not rubbing or massaging affected leg and avoiding injury
  –to wear medical identification.
- For anticoagulation safety, tell the patient to:
  – use an electric razor
  – use a soft toothbrush
  – monitor bruises and call the doctor if they grow.
- Tell the patient to seek help if the following occur:
  – chest pain
  – blood in the sputum
  – difficulty breathing
  – hard, fast breathing
  – pain, warmth, redness, ulceration, or increasing size of involved leg.

DILATED CARDIOMYOPATHY

By far the most common type of cardiomyopathy, dilated cardiomyopathy is a progressive disorder in which the fibers of the heart deteriorate until the heart loses its ability to pump blood effectively. The heart eventually becomes enlarged and rounded. The cause of dilated cardiomyopathy isn't known, but it seems to be linked with excessive alcohol intake, pregnancy, hypertension, and viral infections. If heart contractility doesn't improve with medication, the prognosis is poor.

Symptoms include gradually worsening tiredness, weakness, and chest pain. As the heart fails, the patient may also experience difficulty breathing, a rapid

TEACHING TOPICS

MEDICATIONS

- Thiazide diuretics, potassium-sparing diuretics, and loop diuretics cause excretion of fluid and salt in urine, decreasing heart congestion.
- Potassium supplements replace lost potassium.
- Digitalis glycosides increase the force of ventricular contractions and slow heart rate.
- Angiotensin-converting enzyme inhibitors increase cardiac output by peripheral vasodilation.
- Anticoagulants prevent clot formation.
- Antiarrhythmics help keep the heart rhythm normal and regular.

ACTIVITY

- May be extremely restricted; sometimes bed rest
- No activities that trigger breathing difficulty or extreme tiredness

NUTRITION

- Low-salt diet
- No alcohol

heart rate, palpitations, peripheral edema, enlarged neck veins, and swelling of the liver.

POTENTIAL COMPLICATIONS
- Heart failure
- Arrhythmias
- Emboli

TREATMENTS
- Oxygen
- Implantation of automatic internal cardiac defibrillator (if appropriate)
- Stress reduction and relaxation techniques
- Myocardial transplant in end-stage disease

RISK FACTORS
- Excessive alcohol intake over a long period
- Pregnancy
- Hypertension
- Viral infections

AFTERCARE
- Offer the patient emotional support and (if needed) counseling.
- Tell the patient to wear medical identification.
- For anticoagulation safety, tell the patient to:
  - use an electric razor
  - use a soft toothbrush
  - monitor bruises and call the doctor if they grow.
- Tell the patient to seek help if the following occur:
  - increasing tiredness and weakness
  - chest pain
  - difficulty breathing
  - increasing peripheral edema
  - upper respiratory infection.

ENDOCARDITIS

Endocarditis — sometimes called subacute bacterial endocarditis — is an inflammation of the endocardium, the inside lining of the heart. It results from infection with bacteria, yeast, fungi, or other microbes. The patient typically already has a heart condition, such as valve disease or congenital heart disease; I.V. drug users are also at increased risk.

Signs and symptoms include fever, weakness, appetite loss, headache, and general musculoskeletal aches. The patient may say he feels like he has the flu. Before antibiotics became available, endocarditis was usually fatal.

TEACHING TOPICS

MEDICATIONS

- Antibiotics (such as streptomycin, cefazolin, and penicillins) eradicate the infection.
- Anticoagulants (such as warfarin) prevent clot formation.
- If heart failure occurs, medications for treatment of heart failure may be needed (see "Heart failure," page 44).

ACTIVITY

- Gradually increasing activity with rest periods

NUTRITION

- High-protein diet

POTENTIAL COMPLICATIONS
- Valvular stenosis
- Heart failure
- Arrhythmias
- Emboli, especially in the kidneys, spleen, brain, and lungs
- Myocardial infarction

TREATMENTS
- Continuing antibiotic administration after discharge
- Valve replacement surgery when appropriate

RISK FACTORS
- Preexisting heart condition (such as rheumatic, valvular, or congenital heart disease)
- Medical procedures that disturb the endocardium (such as cardiac surgery, use of a long-term indwelling I.V. catheter)
- I.V. drug use
- Immunosuppression

AFTERCARE
- Tell the patient to:
  – notify all dentists and doctors of endocarditis risk and the need for prophylactic antibiotics
  – wear medical identification
  – stop using oral contraceptives and use another contraceptive while taking antibiotics.
- For anticoagulation safety, tell the patient to:
  – use an electric razor
  – use a soft toothbrush
  – monitor bruises and call the doctor if they grow.
- Tell the patient to seek help if the following occur:
  – chest pain
  – shortness of breath
  – fever
  – chills alternating with sweating
  – extreme tiredness
  – swelling of hands or feet.

HEART FAILURE

In heart failure, the heart can't pump enough blood to meet the body's needs. Heart failure can come on suddenly or build up over years. It results from failure of either the left or right side of the heart, and failure of one side of the heart usually triggers failure of the other side. The left side usually fails first, typically from coronary artery disease (CAD). Left-sided heart failure can also result from hypertension, valvular disease, and cardiomyopathy. When the left side of the heart can't pump out enough blood, the blood collects on the left side of the heart and backs up into the blood vessels of the lungs. This causes shortness of breath, at first only when the patient moves around but eventually even at rest. Other signs can include coughing and wheezing.

TEACHING TOPICS

MEDICATIONS

- Thiazide diuretics, potassium-sparing diuretics, and loop diuretics cause excretion of fluid and salt in urine, decreasing heart congestion.
- Potassium supplements replace lost potassium.
- Digitalis glycosides increase the force of ventricular contractions and slow heart rate.
- Angiotensin-converting enzyme inhibitors increase cardiac output by peripheral vasodilation.
- Anticoagulants prevent clot formation.

ACTIVITY

- As tolerated; activity must stop if fatigue or shortness of breath occur
- Regular, progressive exercise to build up conditioning if possible; not indicated for patients on severe activity restriction or bed rest
- No overexertion or exposure to temperature extremes
- Exertion alternated with rest, paced activities, and no activities that trigger symptoms
- Use of energy-efficient techniques and devices (consultation with occupational therapist)

NUTRITION

- Low-sodium diet; patient should check food labels for hidden salt (in flavorings such as monosodium glutamate and horseradish and in soft drinks, especially diet drinks with saccharin).
- Possible fluid restriction
- Possible increased or decreased potassium in diet (depending on medications)

Right-sided heart failure usually follows left-sided heart failure. Rarely, right-sided heart failure occurs first. When it does, it usually stems from a congenital disorder or cor pulmonale. Right-sided heart failure causes swelling of the feet and ankles, weakness and fatigue, frequent urination, abdominal swelling, liver and spleen enlargement, loss of appetite, nausea and vomiting, and weight gain.

POTENTIAL COMPLICATIONS
- Pulmonary edema
- Pneumonia and other respiratory infections
- Arrhythmias
- Thromboembolism
- Venostasis

TREATMENTS
- Oxygen
- Smoking cessation
- Stress reduction and relaxation techniques
- Elevation of legs to reduce swelling
- Antiembolism stockings
- Heart valve replacement if defective valve is the cause
- Myocardial transplant in end-stage disease

RISK FACTORS
- Family history of cardiovascular disease
- Gender and age (men ages 30 to 55, postmenopausal women and women over 50)
- Congenital heart disorders
- CAD
- Valvular disease
- Smoking
- High serum cholesterol
- Other chronic diseases (such as hypertension and diabetes mellitus)
- Obesity
- Sedentary lifestyle
- Diet high in fat, cholesterol, calories, or salt
- Stress, hostility, and anger

AFTERCARE
- Tell the patient to:
  – watch for sodium in nonprescription medications
  – know indications of digoxin toxicity
  – check weight daily and report sudden or steady gain
  – minimize exposure to infection
  – take and record his pulse
  – wear medical identification
  – use an electric razor
  – use a soft toothbrush
  – monitor bruises.
- Tell him to seek help for:
  – shortness of breath
  – difficulty breathing
  – persistent coughing
  – fast heartbeat
  – occurrence or worsening of peripheral edema
  – loss of appetite
  – increased urination.

HYPERTENSION

Defined as blood pressure consistently above 140/90 mm Hg, hypertension affects nearly a quarter of the population of the United States. Most of the hypertensive population has essential, or primary, hypertension, which has no identifiable cause. Secondary hypertension results from a known underlying cause, such as renal or endocrine disease.

Although some patients may experience headaches early on in the disease, many have no symptoms, making early detection less likely. Later signs and symptoms may include dizziness, numbness, palpitations, vision changes, and nosebleeds.

TEACHING TOPICS

MEDICATIONS

- Antihypertensives reduce blood pressure.
- Beta blockers lower blood pressure, reduce the occurrence of anginal attacks, and control rapid heart rate.
- Calcium channel blockers lower blood pressure and reduce the frequency and severity of chest pain.
- Angiotensin-converting enzyme inhibitors increase cardiac output by peripheral vasodilation.
- Thiazide diuretics, potassium-sparing diuretics, and loop diuretics cause excretion of fluid and salt in urine, decreasing heart congestion.
- Potassium supplements replace lost potassium.

ACTIVITY

- Regular aerobic exercise as tolerated; exercise should stop if dizziness occurs
- No isometric activities (such as straining during a bowel movement, heavy lifting, pushing or pulling)

NUTRITION

- Low-sodium diet if sodium sensitive
- Patient should check food labels for fat and sodium and for hidden salt (in flavorings such as monosodium glutamate and horseradish and in soft drinks, especially diet drinks with saccharin)
- Possible increased or decreased potassium in diet
- Possible increased calcium and decreased caffeine intake
- Supervised dieting for overweight patient
- Limited alcohol intake (up to two drinks per day, as permitted)

Over time, the higher-than-normal pressure of the blood flowing through the circulatory system damages the arteries and capillaries, making them sclerotic, tortuous, and weak. Eventually, not enough blood flows to such key organs as the brain, heart, kidneys, and eyes. This can result in serious damage to or destruction of these organs.

POTENTIAL COMPLICATIONS
- Malignant hypertension
- Left ventricular hypertrophy, possibly with coronary insufficiency
- Myocardial infarction
- Heart failure
- Kidney failure
- Cerebrovascular accidents

TREATMENTS
- Smoking cessation
- Stress reduction and relaxation techniques and biofeedback
- Achieving and maintaining appropriate weight

RISK FACTORS
- Family history of hypertension
- Age (over 50)
- Race (higher incidence in African-Americans)
- Obesity (particularly childhood obesity)
- Stress and anger
- Smoking
- Diet high in salt and saturated fats

AFTERCARE
- Teach the patient or caregiver or both to check and record blood pressure readings and to know when to call the doctor.
- Help the patient adhere to medication schedule and lifestyle changes.
- Work with the patient's doctor to minimize the number of medications the patient must take.
- Tell the patient to seek help if the following occur:
  – headache, particularly occipital headache that occurs in the morning
  – dizziness
  – bleeding from the nose.

MYOCARDIAL INFARCTION

Commonly called a heart attack or coronary, myocardial infarction (MI) is the leading cause of death in the United States. It occurs when narrowing or blockage of a coronary artery prevents sufficient blood from reaching part of the heart. The heart first responds to this decreased blood flow with angina (see "Angina pectoris," page 30), but if blood flow isn't quickly restored, the affected heart muscle can become damaged or necrotic. The scar tissue that forms in place of the damaged tissue can't contract the way normal heart tissue does, which compromises circulation. The severity of an MI depends on how much heart muscle was deprived of blood and for how long.

TEACHING TOPICS

MEDICATIONS

- Thrombolytic agents aid in coronary reperfusion.
- Antiarrhythmics treat arrhythmias.
- Antiplatelets slow blood clotting.
- Beta blockers lower blood pressure, reduce the occurrence of anginal attacks, and control rapid heart rate.
- Nitrates prevent or lessen anginal pain.
- Angiotensin-converting enzyme inhibitors increase cardiac output by peripheral vasodilation.

ACTIVITY

- Regular aerobic exercise as tolerated; exercise should stop if chest pain occurs
- No isometric activities (such as straining during a bowel movement, heavy lifting, pushing or pulling)

NUTRITION

- Low-fat, low-sodium diet with limited caffeine intake to lower blood pressure
- Patient should check food labels for fat and sodium content
- Preferred cooking methods: broiling, microwaving, grilling, and roasting
- Supervised dieting for overweight patient
- Limited alcohol intake (up to two drinks per day, as permitted)

Although an MI typically results from coronary artery disease, coronary artery spasm or thrombosis can also trigger an MI. The hallmark is tremendous chest pain unrelieved by nitrates, often radiating down the left shoulder and arm to the hand. Sometimes it also radiates to the right shoulder, up to the neck and jaw, or to the lower chest (mimicking indigestion or heartburn). Other signs and symptoms include shortness of breath, anxiety, sweating, nausea and vomiting, and weakness.

POTENTIAL COMPLICATIONS
- Arrhythmias
- Cardiogenic shock
- Additional MIs
- Heart failure

TREATMENTS
- Smoking cessation
- Stress reduction and relaxation techniques
- Cardiac rehabilitation program
- Percutaneous transluminal angioplasty, stent placement during atherectomy, or coronary artery bypass graft surgery, as appropriate, to provide adequate coronary perfusion

RISK FACTORS
- Family history of cardiovascular disease.
- Gender and age (men ages 30 to 55, postmenopausal women and women over age 50)
- Smoking
- High serum cholesterol
- Other chronic diseases (such as hypertension, diabetes mellitus)
- Obesity
- Sedentary lifestyle
- Diet high in fat, cholesterol, calories, or salt
- Stress, hostility, and anger

AFTERCARE
- Suggest that family members take a cardiopulmonary resuscitation course.
- Teach the patient how to manage anginal pain.
- Tell the patient to seek help if the following occur:
  – chest pain (crushing, tightness, or aching)
  – pain or discomfort in neck, jaw, throat, shoulders, back, or arms
  – nausea, severe indigestion, or heartburn
  – difficulty breathing, weakness, sweating, or dizziness.

PERICARDITIS

Pericarditis is an inflammation of the pericardium, the protective sac that surrounds the heart. Normally, pericardial fluid fills the narrow space between the visceral layer of the pericardium that adheres to the heart and the parietal layer that lines the fibrous pericardium, allowing the heart to contract and move without friction. When the pericardium becomes inflamed, it thickens, scars, and becomes fibrotic, which can constrict the heart.

Pericarditis can occur in acute and progressive, chronic forms. It can result from various causes, including viral, fungal, or bacterial infections (such as tuberculosis); damage to the heart from myocardial infarction, surgery, or trauma; malignant tumors; autoimmune diseases; drug reactions; and radiation therapy.

TEACHING TOPICS

MEDICATIONS

- Antibiotics (such as streptomycin, cefazolin, and penicillins) eradicate the infection.
- Nonsteroidal anti-inflammatory drugs (such as aspirin and indomethacin) relieve pain and inflammation.
- Steroids (such as prednisone) decrease inflammation and pain.
- If heart failure occurs, medications for treatment of heart failure may be needed (see "Heart failure," page 44).

ACTIVITY

- Gradually increasing activity with rest periods
- Possible limitations on strenuous activities

NUTRITION

- Low-fat, low-cholesterol diet (slows progression of coronary artery disease)
- Nutrition guidelines for heart failure if heart failure occurs (see "Heart failure," page 44)

Signs and symptoms include pain, anxiety, fever, difficulty breathing, distended neck veins, delayed capillary refill time, and swelling of the abdomen and legs.

POTENTIAL COMPLICATIONS
- Heart failure secondary to cardiac constriction
- Pleural effusion
- Cardiac tamponade

Treatments
- Achieving and maintaining appropriate weight
- Pericardiectomy if medication proves ineffective

Risk factors
- Damage to the heart from myocardial infarction, surgery, or trauma
- Autoimmune diseases
- Viral, fungal, or bacterial infections
- Malignant tumors
- Drug reactions
- Radiation therapy

Aftercare
- Tell the patient to:
  – minimize exposure to infection
  – stop using oral contraceptives (if applicable) and use another contraceptive while taking antibiotics.
- Tell the patient to seek help if the following occur:
  – chest pain (crushing, tightness, or aching)
  – pain or discomfort in neck, jaw, throat, shoulders, back, or arms
  – nausea
  – fever
  – sore throat
  – upper respiratory infection.

PERIPHERAL ARTERIAL OCCLUSIVE DISEASE

Peripheral arterial occlusive disease occurs when arteries can't deliver enough blood to the tissues they supply. It can be acute or chronic. Chronic disease — the most common type — occurs when fatty plaques build up on arterial walls (atherosclerosis), narrowing the arteries and sometimes causing stenosis, frequently at bifurcations of the arteries. Acute disease results from a sudden decrease in blood flow from a thrombus, embolus, vasospasm, inflammation, or trauma.

Because the lower extremities are more prone to atherosclerosis than the upper extremities, signs and symptoms of peripheral arterial occlusive disease usually occur in the legs. Initial signs include intermittent claudication in one or both

---

TEACHING TOPICS

MEDICATIONS

- Anticoagulants (such as warfarin) prevent further clot formation.
- Hemorrheologics (such as pentoxifylline) reduce blood viscosity and microcirculatory flow for better tissue oxygenation.

ACTIVITY

- Regular aerobic exercise

NUTRITION

- Diet low in salt, cholesterol, and saturated fat
- Adequate protein
- Foods high in vitamins B and C

limbs. As the disease progresses, pain may occur at rest, even waking the patient from sleep.

The skin on the legs may feel cool to the touch, although the patient may feel as if his skin is burning. He may also feel tingling or numbness. The skin may look shiny and slightly to very pale (when the legs are elevated) or darkish red (when the legs are in a dependent position). Other signs include diminished or absent pedal pulses and sparse hair growth on the legs. In the later stages, the legs may ulcerate or become gangrenous.

POTENTIAL COMPLICATIONS
- Severe ischemia
- Skin ulcerations
- Gangrene
- Emboli

TREATMENTS
- Regular exercise program
- Achieving and maintaining appropriate weight
- Skin and foot care
- Smoking cessation
- Stress management and relaxation techniques and biofeedback
- Endarterectomy, bypass grafting, atherectomy, transluminal or laser angioplasty, stenting, or amputation, as appropriate, if medical treatment isn't effective

RISK FACTORS
- Smoking
- Hypertension
- Diabetes mellitus
- Obesity
- Hyperlipidemia

AFTERCARE
- Tell the patient not to use adhesive tape on affected areas.
- Tell the patient to seek help if the following occur:
  – sudden, extreme pain
  – difficulty breathing
  – change in color of affected area
  – no pulse in affected leg or arm
  – loss of movement in affected leg or arm.

RAYNAUD'S PHENOMENON

Affecting more women than men, Raynaud's phenomenon is characterized by spasms of the arterioles that are triggered by cold or stress. These spasms restrict blood flow to the hands and fingers. The condition is associated with autoimmune disorders, such as scleroderma, systemic lupus erythematosus, and rheumatoid arthritis. Because indications of Raynaud's phenomenon may appear years before signs and symptoms of any associated autoimmune disorder, patients with the disorder should also be thoroughly assessed for autoimmune disease.

When spasms of the arterioles occur, the fingers blanch and may become numb. Tissue hypoxia then causes local vasodilation, and the fingers look bluish because of the presence of deoxygenated blood. After the spasms stop and normal

TEACHING TOPICS

MEDICATIONS

- Calcium channel blockers (such as nifedipine) cause peripheral vasodilation.
- Antihypertensives (such as prazosin) inhibit peripheral vasoconstriction.

ACTIVITY

- Extra precautions to protect hands as necessary (wearing gloves for winter sports, performing such activities as typing or playing a piano in a warm setting)

NUTRITION

- Possibly limited caffeine intake (because of its vasoconstrictive effect)

blood flow resumes, the fingers become red and may throb. An episode can last anywhere from a few minutes to several hours and may occur either unilaterally or bilaterally. Spasms can also affect the feet and toes and, very rarely, the ears, nose, and cheeks.

POTENTIAL COMPLICATIONS
- Carpal tunnel syndrome
- Gangrene of the fingertips (rare)

TREATMENTS
- Smoking cessation
- Stress management and relaxation techniques
- Biofeedback to teach patients to increase hand temperature
- Cervical sympathectomy as appropriate

RISK FACTORS
- Gender (incidence higher in women)
- Climate (incidence higher in cold, damp locales)
- Arteriosclerosis
- Autoimmune disorders (such as scleroderma, systemic lupus erythematosus, rheumatoid arthritis)
- Exposure to vinyl chloride

AFTERCARE
- Tell the patient to:
  - take extra care to prevent cuts and burns if the hands become numb
  - understand that birth control pills and medications that contain ergot (such as ergotamine tartrate) can trigger episodes of vasoconstriction.
  - notify all dentists and doctors about Raynaud's phenomenon so they can avoid inappropriate medications and treatments.
- Tell the patient to seek help if increasingly frequent or severe attacks occur.

VALVULAR HEART DISEASE

Normally, heart valves allow sufficient blood to flow through the heart in one direction only. In valvular heart disease, a malfunctioning valve can slow blood flow or allow some blood to flow backward. When a valve malfunctions, the heart tries to compensate; if the heart can't pump enough blood through the circulatory system, heart failure may occur.

Valvular heart disease can result from a congenitally abnormal heart valve. It can also stem from inflammatory heart disease (such as rheumatic fever or endocarditis) that damages the valve or from calcification of the valve (in older patients).

TEACHING TOPICS

MEDICATIONS

- Diuretics cause excretion of fluid and salt in urine, decreasing heart congestion.
- Potassium supplements replace lost potassium.
- Digitalis glycosides increase force of ventricular contractions and slow heart rate.
- Beta blockers lower blood pressure, reduce the occurrence of anginal attacks, and control rapid heart rate.
- Antiarrhythmics help to keep the heart rhythm normal and regular.
- Angiotensin-converting enzyme inhibitors increase cardiac output by peripheral vasodilation.
- Anticoagulants prevent clot formation.
- Nitrates prevent or lessen anginal pain.

ACTIVITY

- Normal activity unless symptoms occur
- No activities that bring on difficulty in breathing or extreme tiredness
- Severely limited activity with certain types of valvular disease (as ordered by doctor)

NUTRITION

- Possibly low-salt diet

A malfunctioning heart valve can be heard as a murmur. Other signs and symptoms include tiring easily, shortness of breath, chest pain, faintness, and peripheral edema, although some patients have no signs or symptoms. Signs and symptoms may come on suddenly or gradually, and the patient may first be seen in heart failure.

POTENTIAL COMPLICATIONS
- Endocarditis
- Cardiac hypertrophy
- Heart failure
- Arrhythmias
- Emboli

TREATMENTS
- Smoking cessation
- Wound care
- Surgical valve repair or replacement, as appropriate, if medical treatment is ineffective

RISK FACTORS
- Inflammatory heart disease (such as rheumatic fever or endocarditis)
- Age (calcification of valves in older patients)

AFTERCARE
- Tell the patient to:
  – notify all dentists and doctors of endocarditis risk and the need for prophylactic antibiotics
  – wear medical identification.
- For anticoagulation safety, tell the patient to:
  – use an electric razor
  – use a soft toothbrush
  – monitor bruises and call the doctor if they grow.
- Tell the patient to seek help if the following occur:
  – difficulty breathing
  – increasing tiredness
  – irregular heartbeats
  – hard, fast heartbeats
  – dizziness
  – fainting
  – chest pain.

ASTHMA

Asthma is the hyperreactive response of bronchial airways to certain stimuli that leads to inflammation, swelling, and airway constriction. Mucus plugs can impede airflow still further, making it increasingly difficult for the patient to breathe. Other signs and symptoms of asthma include severe wheezing and unrelenting cough. An attack is usually reversible (spontaneously or with treatment) but can rapidly escalate to status asthmaticus and death.

Incidence is on the rise in the United States and, despite better drugs and treatments, morbidity and the mortality are also increasing. Many of the deaths that occur during attacks could be prevented if patients learned the early signs and symptoms of an attack so that they could seek out and receive prompt treatment.

TEACHING TOPICS

MEDICATIONS

- Bronchodilators (such as albuterol, aminophylline, isoproterenol, terbutaline, and theophylline) open airways, making breathing easier.
- Anticholinergic bronchodilators (such as ipratropium) block acetylcholine.
- Steroids (such as beclomethasone, flunisolide, and prednisone) decrease inflammation and swelling in airways.
- Mast cell stabilizers (such as cromolyn and nedocromil) help prevent attacks by decreasing airway reactivity to allergens.
- Antibiotics (such as amoxicillin and ampicillin) treat respiratory infections, if necessary.

ACTIVITY

- Regular aerobic exercise
- No overexertion; alternating activity with rest
- Limited activity during weather extremes and when ozone levels are high

NUTRITION

- Healthy diet based on recommended portions from the food pyramid
- Small, frequent meals (may be better tolerated)
- Adequate hydration

The hyperactive response that triggers an attack seems to result from an interaction between genetics and environment; specific triggers vary with each patient. Triggers can be immunologic (pollen, smoke, fumes, dust, and weather changes) or nonimmunologic (viral infections and exercise), and strong emotions can exacerbate an attack. Onset of the disorder usually occurs before adolescence but can occur at any age.

POTENTIAL COMPLICATIONS
- Status asthmaticus
- Respiratory arrest
- Pneumonia

TREATMENTS

- Smoking cessation and avoiding second-hand smoke
- Medications (antibiotics, bronchodilators, corticosteroids) administered orally or by nebulizer or metered-dose inhaler
- Oxygen therapy
- Breathing exercises (pursed-lip breathing)
- Stress management and relaxation techniques and biofeedback
- Humidifier

RISK FACTORS

- Gender (higher incidence in males)
- Race (higher incidence in blacks)

AFTERCARE

- Teach the patient (and the caregiver) how to identify and eliminate or manage triggers.
- Tell the patient to:
  – avoid taking over-the-counter drugs without doctor's approval
  – avoid crowds and people with infections.
- Tell the patient to seek help if he has:
  – a severe attack that can't be quickly controlled
  – fever during an attack
  – chest pain
  – shortness of breath unrelated to exercise or coughing.

BRONCHITIS

Sometimes called tracheobronchitis, bronchitis is an inflammation of the mucous membranes of the trachea and bronchi. It typically develops after a viral upper respiratory infection (from a rhinovirus or an adenovirus) although it can also develop after a bacterial respiratory infection (from a hemophilus or streptococcus organism or from *Mycoplasma pneumoniae*). Inhaling irritating chemicals or gases, aspirating food or other objects, and overzealously suctioning the trachea can also cause bronchitis.

Signs and symptoms include midsternal chest pain, sore throat, fever, headache, general achy discomfort, and (initially) dry cough. As the inflamma-

TEACHING TOPICS

MEDICATIONS

- Antibiotics (such as amoxicillin, cefaclor, co-trimoxazole, erythromycin, and tetracycline) combat bacterial infections.
- Antipyretics (such as aspirin and acetaminophen) reduce fever.
- Bronchodilators (such as terbutaline) open airways, making breathing easier.
- Steroids, systemic or inhaled (such as prednisone and beclomethasone), decrease inflammation and swelling in airways.
- Anticholinergics (such as dicyclomine) relax smooth muscle and relieve spasms.
- Cough suppressants (such as codeine, hydrocodone, and dextromethorphan) suppress a nonproductive cough.

ACTIVITY

- Rest until fever subsides, in acute brochitis
- Possible limited activity to promote healing and help prevent exacerbation
- No exposure to cold air (may worsen pain)

NUTRITION

- Healthy diet based on recommended portions from the food pyramid
- Increased fluids (to maintain hydration)
- No alcohol (alcohol suppresses upper airway reflexes)

tion progresses, the cough may become productive and sputum may become thick, purulent, and (occasionally) blood tinged. The cough may linger for 2 to 3 weeks after other symptoms have subsided.

POTENTIAL COMPLICATIONS
- Pneumonia
- Chronic obstructive pulmonary disease (from chronic bronchitis)

Treatments

- Effective coughing techniques (including splinting to ease discomfort)
- Humidifier use
- Smoking cessation and avoiding second-hand smoke
- Treatment of associated disorders such as gastroesophageal reflux disease

Risk factors

- Respiratory infections
- Inhaling caustic or toxic chemicals or pollutants
- Aspirating food or other objects

Aftercare

- Tell the patient to:
  – avoid spreading infection by sneezing or coughing into a tissue, disposing of used tissues properly, and washing hands frequently
  – stop using oral contraceptives (if applicable) and use another contraceptive while taking antibiotics (antibiotics can prevent oral contraceptives from working).
- Tell the patient to seek help if the following occur:
  – recurring fever
  – purulent or blood-tinged sputum
  – worsening chest pain
  – worsening cough.

CHRONIC OBSTRUCTIVE PULMONARY DISEASE

Chronic obstructive pulmonary disease (COPD) is a combination of conditions—specifically, chronic bronchitis, emphysema, and chronic asthma. The most common predisposing factor is smoking; other factors include chronic upper respiratory infections and exposure to environmental and occupational dust (such as asbestos) and gases.

COPD results in inflamed, narrowed airways; increased mucus production (from chronic bronchitis); decreased lung elasticity; and alveolar destruction (from emphysema). Bronchospasms (from asthma) obstruct airflow and impair gas exchange.

If chronic bronchitis is the primary underlying disease, the patient typically has a productive cough and may have decreased exercise tolerance, dyspnea, pe-

TEACHING TOPICS

MEDICATIONS

- Bronchodilators open airways, making breathing easier.
- Antihistamines help limit airway constriction, making breathing easier.
- Steroids decrease inflammation and swelling in airways.
- Expectorants make mucus thinner and easier to cough up.
- Mast cell stabilizers decrease airway reactivity to allergens, helping to prevent attacks.
- Antibiotics prevent or treat respiratory infections

ACTIVITY

- Progressive walking program
- Alternating activity with rest to avoid fatigue
- Energy-conservation measures (such as sitting to bathe and shave), with possible occupational therapy consult
- Limited activity when ozone levels are high
- No exposure to cold air (may trigger bronchospasms)

NUTRITION

- Increased calories in diet
- High-protein, low-carbohydrate diet
- Increased fluids (to maintain hydration)
- Small, frequent meals (may be better tolerated)
- Resting before and after meals if shortness of breath interferes with eating

ripheral edema, and cyanosis. He is likely to have a normal chest diameter and be overweight.

When emphysema is the primary disease, the patient typically complains of dyspnea on exertion and, eventually, at rest. The patient may be thin and, because he hyperventilates in an attempt to offset hypoxemia, he may look pink. He typically has a barrel chest.

When asthma is the primary component, the patient typically complains of dyspnea, wheezing, and sometimes coughing.

POTENTIAL COMPLICATIONS
- Respiratory infections (such as influenza and pneumonia)
- Cor pulmonale
- Acute respiratory failure
- Pneumothorax

TREATMENTS
- Smoking cessation
- Breathing exercises (diaphragmatic and pursed-lip breathing)
- Bronchial hygiene (postural drainage, adequate hydration)
- Low-flow oxygen therapy
- Stress management and relaxation techniques
- Oxygen, nebulizer
- Lung volume reduction surgery for some patients, primarily those with emphysema

RISK FACTORS
- Smoking cigarettes (80% to 90% of all cases)
- Gender and age (higher incidence in men over age 45)
- Race (higher incidence in whites)
- Environmental and occupational dust and gases
- Chronic upper respiratory infections
- Genetic predisposition

AFTERCARE
- Teach the patient (and the caregiver) to identify and eliminate or manage triggers.
- Tell the patient to:
  – consider wearing medical identification
  – avoid crowds and people with infections
  – keep the house warm and humidified.
- Tell the patient to seek help if he experiences:
  – respiratory infection
  – increased difficulty breathing
  – increased production or change in color of sputum
  – change in coughing pattern
  – fever
  – sore throat
  – GI symptoms (including blood in stool).

CYSTIC FIBROSIS

Cystic fibrosis (CF) is a chronic, progressive congenital disease that was once considered a pediatric disorder because patients rarely reached adulthood. More recently, patients have lived into their 30s, even 40s.

CF is usually detected at birth, although symptoms may not be noticeable until months or years later. The disease results from dysfunction of the exocrine glands, which produce abnormally thick, sticky mucus.

Although CF affects several body systems, it most severely affects the pulmonary system. The cilia can't clear the thick mucus, resulting in plugged airways and pockets of mucus that foster infection and ultimately resulting in restrictive lung disease. Sweat glands affected by the disease produce abnormally salty sweat. In the digestive system, thick mucus can block pancreatic ducts, prevent-

---

TEACHING TOPICS

MEDICATIONS

- Bronchodilators open airways and improve breathing.
- Mast cell stabilizers help prevent bronchospasm by decreasing airway reactivity to allergens.
- Steroids decrease inflammation and swelling in airways.
- Antibiotics prevent or treat respiratory infections.
- Pancreatic enzyme supplements help digest food.
- Vitamin and iron supplements replace those not absorbed by digestive tract.
- Digoxin increases ventricular contraction force if pulmonary hypertension and cor pulmonale develop.

ACTIVITY

- Regular aerobic exercise, with breathing treatments before exercise and adequate hydration and salt supplements as needed during exercise
- No exercise on hot days or when ozone levels are high

NUTRITION

- Diet high in calories, salt, protein, and fat
- Vitamin supplements (especially A, D, E, and K)
- Pancreatic enzyme supplements (when consuming carbohydrates and fats)

ing the delivery of digestive enzymes to the intestines, which results in malabsorption and large, foul-smelling, pale, fatty stools. In the male reproductive system, mucus can clog the vas deferens, preventing sperm from getting through (the vas deferens may also be anatomically malformed); in the female reproductive system, cervical mucus may not allow passage of sperm. Pregnancy can exacerbate CF, although most patients with the disease are infertile.

POTENTIAL COMPLICATIONS
- Pulmonary disorders (atelectasis, pneumonia, pneumothorax, cor pulmonale, hemoptysis, respiratory infection, and respiratory failure)
- GI disorders (dehydration, intestinal obstruction, esophageal varices, and cirrhosis)

TREATMENTS
- Oxygen therapy
- Nebulizer use
- Medications (antibiotics, bronchodilators, pulmonary enzymes, mucolytics) administered orally or by nebulizer or metered-dose inhaler
- Bronchial hygiene (postural drainage, percussion, vibration, coughing, adequate hydration)
- Breathing exercises (forced expiratory breathing)

RISK FACTORS
- Race (higher incidence in whites)
- Genetic predisposition (autosomal recessive disorder)

AFTERCARE
- Offer the patient and family teaching and emotional support; suggest counseling or national or local support groups.
- For the adult patient, discuss reproductive sterility and offer genetic counseling.
- Tell the patient to receive pneumonia vaccinations every 10 years and yearly flu vaccinations.
- Tell the patient to seek help if he has:
  – increased thickness of or blood in sputum
  – fever
  – weight loss
  – unusual tiredness
  – loss of appetite
  – more fatty stools than usual.

INFLUENZA

Although people commonly use the term "flu" to refer to many upper respiratory conditions, true influenza is an inflammatory response to infection of the airway by myxovirus A, B, or C. In the United States, influenza occurs mainly in the winter months and tends to be epidemic. It affects all age-groups but poses the greatest risk to the very young, the elderly, those with chronic disorders, and the debilitated. Transmission occurs by breathing in droplets that contain the myxovirus or by touching infected people or contaminated items. The virus can live for 2 to 3 days on objects, making hand washing especially important during flu season. Patients are contagious before symptoms appear and remain contagious for about 3 days.

The hallmarks of the flu include a sudden onset of fever (usually over 102° F [38.9° C]), aching muscles throughout the body, and cough. Some patients also have a headache, sore throat, and runny nose. The flu usually subsides in less

TEACHING TOPICS

MEDICATIONS
- Antivirals combat viral infections.
- Antipyretics reduce fever.
- Analgesics relieve headache and muscle pain.
- Antihistamines dry up watery eyes and runny nose.
- Decongestants cause vasoconstriction of nasal mucous membranes, relieving congestion.
- Cough suppressants decrease the cough reflex.
- Expectorants make mucus thinner and easier to cough up.
- Antibiotics eradicate secondary bacterial infections.

ACTIVITY
- Bed rest during the acute phase
- Gradual return to normal activity (to limit the risk of developing a secondary infection)

NUTRITION
- Increased fluids (to maintain hydration)

than 1 week, although the patient may feel tired for much longer. The real dangers lie in the possibility of such secondary infections as viral or bacterial pneumonia and in the effects of dehydration in high-risk patients.

The particular strain of myxovirus changes from year to year, so the appropriate flu vaccine should be administered each year at least 2 weeks before the start of flu season. Immunity lasts no more than 6 months. Yearly vaccines should be obtained by health care professionals (due to exposure to the virus), the elderly, and chronically ill and debilitated patients. Young children over 6 months may receive a split dose.

POTENTIAL COMPLICATIONS
- Viral or bacterial pneumonia
- Bronchitis
- Acute sinusitis
- Otitis media

TREATMENTS
- Humidifier use
- Smoking cessation

RISK FACTORS
- Chronic illness
- General debilitation
- Crowded living conditions or institutional living
- Working in a health care setting

AFTERCARE
- Tell the patient:
  – who has had Guillain-Barré syndrome or is allergic to eggs that he should not receive the flu vaccine
  – at high risk to get annual flu vaccine before start of flu season
  – to avoid spreading infection by sneezing or coughing into tissue, disposing of used tissues properly, and washing hands often
  – to avoid crowds and people with respiratory infections.
- Tell the patient to seek help if:
  – symptoms worsen or don't improve in a week
  – dehydration occurs.

PNEUMONIA

Still one of the leading causes of death in the United States despite new vaccines and treatments, pneumonia is an acute inflammation of the lungs that impairs gas exchange. Several precipitating factors can cause the inflammation, including bacteria (such as streptococcus, klebsiella, staphylococcus, haemophilus, and legionella), viruses (such as influenza, adenovirus, respiratory syncytial virus, rubeola, varicella, and cytomegalovirus), mycoplasmas (such as *Mycoplasma pneumoniae*), fungi (such as aspergillus), and protozoa (such as *Pneumocystis carinii*). Other causes include aspiration of food, fluid, or vomitus and inhalation of chemicals, smoke, or dust. Depending on the cause, pneumonia may or may not be infectious.

The onset of pneumonia typically causes fever, shaking chills, sweating, pleuritic pain, difficulty breathing, coughing, and unusual tiredness, although elderly

TEACHING TOPICS

MEDICATIONS

- Antibiotics (such as amoxicillin, cefaclor, nafcillin, cotrimoxazole, clindamycin, and erythromycin) eradicate bacterial infections.
- Antifungals (such as flucytosine) eradicate fungal infections.
- Antiprotozoals (such as pentamidine) combat protozoal infections.
- Antivirals (such as amantadine) combat viral infections.
- Antipyretics (such as aspirin and acetaminophen) reduce fever.

ACTIVITY

- Alternating activity with rest to prevent overexertion
- Gradual return to normal activity (to limit the risk of a recurrence)

NUTRITION

- Healthy diet based on recommended portions from the food pyramid
- Adequate hydration

patients may first present with disorientation or dehydration. Most patients can receive treatment at home; patients with severe pneumonia and very young, elderly, immunocompromised, or debilitated patients may need hospitalization. Recurrences of the disease can cause progressive damage to the lungs and vulnerability to further illness.

POTENTIAL COMPLICATIONS
- Atelectasis
- Empyema
- Adult respiratory distress syndrome
- Respiratory failure
- Pericarditis, endocarditis, or meningitis
- Lung abscesses

TREATMENTS
- Smoking cessation
- Oxygen therapy
- Bronchial hygiene (postural drainage, percussion, vibration, therapeutic coughing)
- Breathing exercises (diaphragmatic and pursed-lip breathing)

RISK FACTORS
- Age (children under age 1 and adults over age 65)
- Upper respiratory infection
- Smoking
- Chronic lung disease
- Immunosuppression
- Prolonged bed rest

AFTERCARE
- Tell the patient to:
  – receive pneumonia and flu vaccines the following year
  – avoid spreading infection by sneezing or coughing into a tissue, disposing of used tissues properly, and washing hands frequently
  – avoid crowds and people with respiratory infections.
- Tell the patient to seek help if the following occur:
  – fever
  – sweating
  – difficulty breathing
  – persistent coughing
  – upper respiratory infection.

PULMONARY EMBOLISM

Pulmonary embolism results when a dislodged thrombus or other material lodges in the pulmonary blood vessels, impeding blood flow. The embolus typically comes from thrombi in the deep veins of the legs—usually from above the knee—or pelvis. The embolus may consist of blood (from a thrombus); less common types include fat, air, bone marrow, amniotic fluid, other types of tissue fragments, and (occasionally) foreign objects, such as a catheter tip. Emboli vary in size, from tiny to fairly large, and in number, from only one to many.

Signs and symptoms include difficulty breathing, rapid heart rate, and chest pain. The severity and onset of symptoms depend on the size and number of the emboli and the amount of lung tissue affected. Severe, sudden symptoms may mimic those of a myocardial infarction; however, the pain from pulmonary em-

TEACHING TOPICS

MEDICATIONS

- Anticoagulants (such as heparin and warfarin) prevent blood clots.
- Thrombolytic enzymes (such as streptokinase) dissolve existing clots.

ACTIVITY

- No overexertion; alternating activity with rest
- Regular walking program
- No sitting with legs crossed; legs should be elevated
- No sitting or standing for long periods

NUTRITION

- Diet low in vitamin K
- Adequate food and fluid intake

bolism is worse on inhalation. The patient may feel restless and anxious from hypoxemia, which develops when a portion of the lungs is ventilated but not perfused. Other signs and symptoms include coughing, a feeling of faintness, and blood in the sputum. Pulmonary embolism causes over 50,000 deaths a year, more than half within 2 hours of the event.

POTENTIAL COMPLICATIONS
- Extension or recurrence of pulmonary embolism
- Pulmonary hypertension
- Atelectasis
- Right-sided heart failure and decreased cardiac output
- Shock
- Cardiopulmonary arrest

TREATMENTS
- No garments that bind legs or obstruct circulation
- Oxygen therapy
- Smoking cessation and avoiding second-hand smoke
- No tobacco use

RISK FACTORS
- Venostasis
- Fractures
- Increased blood coagulability
- Abdominal, vascular, or hip surgery
- Thrombophlebitis
- Atrial fibrillation
- Obesity
- Pregnancy
- Use of oral contraceptives

AFTERCARE
- Tell the patient on anticoagulant therapy to avoid taking:
  – over-the-counter medications without the doctor's approval
  – salicylates, nonsteroidal anti-inflammatory drugs, cimetidine, and trimethaphan
  – antacids, diuretics, oral contraceptives, and barbiturates.
- Tell the patient to seek help if the following occur:
  – sudden, sharp chest pain
  – difficulty breathing
  – coughing up blood
  – fever
  – calf pain or swelling.

SARCOIDOSIS

Sarcoidosis is an inflammatory disorder that results in the development of granulomatous lesions. The location of the lesions depends on which organs are affected, most commonly the lungs. But granulomas can also develop on other organs, including the lymphatic system, skin, liver, spleen, eyes, bones, salivary glands, joints, and heart.

Although the cause of sarcoidosis isn't known, it's thought to be an immune response to a genetic, infectious, immunologic, or toxic trigger. This immune response causes granulomas to develop on the affected part.

Granulomas that develop on the skin and other obvious places allow ready detection of the disease; other granulomas may only be detected by chance—for in-

---

TEACHING TOPICS

MEDICATIONS

- Steroids, systemic or topical, reduce inflammation and swelling.
- Eyedrops (such as methylcellulose eyedrops) sooth the eyes (if affected).
- Antiarrhythmics (such as digoxin, procainamide, propranolol, quinidine, and verapamil) help keep heart rhythm normal and regular.
- Calcium-chelating agents (such as sodium edetate) bind calcium, promoting calcium excretion.
- Anti-inflammatory agents (such as nonsteroidal anti-inflammatory drugs) decrease inflammation and swelling.
- Vitamin D supplements promote absorption and use of calcium and phosphate.

ACTIVITY

- No overexertion; alternating activity with rest

NUTRITION

- Low-salt, low-potassium, low-calcium diet
- Small, frequent meals (may be better tolerated)
- Adequate hydration

stance, when an asymptomatic patient is being X-rayed for another reason. Other signs and symptoms vary with the location of the lesions and may include a persistent nonproductive cough, shortness of breath, unusual tiredness, fever, pain in the joints, blurred vision, and weight loss. Granulomas can shrink either spontaneously or with treatment. If granulomas on the lungs increase in size, they can result in fibrosis of the lungs and restrictive lung disease.

POTENTIAL COMPLICATIONS
- Pulmonary fibrosis
- Cor pulmonale

TREATMENTS
- Bronchial hygiene (postural drainage)
- Breathing exercises (diaphragmatic breathing)
- Energy-conservation measures, with possible occupational therapy consult

RISK FACTORS
- Race and gender (higher incidence in blacks, particularly women)
- Age (adults ages 20 to 40)

AFTERCARE
- Tell the patient taking a corticosteroid to:
  - avoid stopping the medication suddenly
  - receive regular medical checkups for hypertension, diabetes mellitus, hypokalemia, and development of Cushing's syndrome
  - immediately report indications of infection or GI bleeding.
- Tell the patient to seek help if the following occur:
  - shortness of breath
  - red, watery eyes
  - increasing tiredness
  - fever
  - chest pain
  - joint swelling
  - dizziness.

SLEEP APNEA SYNDROME

Sleep apnea syndrome is a respiratory disorder in which the patient stops breathing for short periods during sleep. A patient is diagnosed with sleep apnea syndrome if he has apneic episodes that last 10 seconds or longer and occur at least 5 times an hour, although apneic episodes can last up to 2 minutes and occur over 100 times a night. Sleep apnea syndrome affects over 1% of the population of the United States and plays a part in many accidents involving motor vehicles and machinery. It can also interfere with a person's ability to work effectively and can affect personality.

A patient can have either obstructive or central nervous system apnea or both types together. The more common type, obstructive sleep apnea, results when the tongue or oropharyngeal tissues partially or completely obstruct the upper airway. In a typical episode, the patient snores increasingly loudly, stops snoring for

TEACHING TOPICS

MEDICATIONS

- Thyroid replacement drugs (such as levothyroxine) improve upper airway patency of patients with hypothyroidism.

ACTIVITY

- Adjusting activities around periods of drowsiness and wakefulness to minimize disruption
- No potentially dangerous activities (such as driving) while drowsy

NUTRITION

- Supervised, safe dieting for overweight patient
- No alcohol (depresses respiratory effort)

a short time, and partially awakens with a loud, violent gasp. A night of such episodes leaves the patient feeling tired and sleep deprived the next day. The typical patient is an obese, middle-aged man with a short, thick neck who snores heavily.

The less common type, central nervous system apnea results from the brain's failure to signal respiratory inhalation. This type of apnea may stem from a stroke or other brain lesion.

POTENTIAL COMPLICATIONS
- Pulmonary hypertension
- Cor pulmonale
- Arrhythmias
- Heart failure

TREATMENTS
- Continuous positive airway pressure (CPAP) or bilevel positive airway pressure (BIPAP)
- Oral appliance that holds jaw forward and keeps upper airway open
- Sleeping on side, not back (pillows or a tennis ball slipped into a pocket sewn onto the back center of a nightshirt help patient stay off back)
- Tracheostomy or craniofacial surgery, if necessary, for patients with severe obstructive sleep apnea

RISK FACTORS
- Obesity
- Gender (higher incidence in men; incidence increases in women after menopause)

AFTERCARE
- Tell the patient to:
  – avoid driving, using power tools, operating heavy machinery, or performing other dangerous activities when drowsy
  – inform all doctors including anesthetists and dentists of his condition
  – wear medical identification
  – receive regular blood pressure assessments.
- Tell the patient to seek help if the following occur:
  – increased daytime sleepiness
  – inability to use CPAP, BIPAP mask, or other equipment
  – CPAP or BIPAP become ineffective.

TUBERCULOSIS

Once fairly well controlled in the United States, the incidence of tuberculosis (TB)—including more virulent forms of the disease—is on the rise. This resurgence is due to a rise in AIDS cases, an influx of immigrants from developing countries with high TB rates, and multidrug-resistant strains (most likely due to TB patients who don't comply with treatment).

TB primarily affects the lungs. Transmission occurs by breathing in droplets that contain the causative agent *Mycobacterium tuberculosis*, although a healthy person must have frequent and close contact with an infected person to acquire the disease. If a person harbors the bacilli in his lungs but doesn't develop symptoms and has normal chest X-rays and negative blood tests, he has TB infection without active disease. If his immune system doesn't destroy the bacilli, they may lie dormant, possibly for years, and may reactivate if he becomes immunocompromised.

Active TB usually affects the lungs first but can disseminate to other vascular organs and areas, including the heart, kidneys, meninges, and bone joints. Signs and symptoms of active TB in the lungs include a persistent cough, night sweats,

TEACHING TOPICS

MEDICATIONS

- Antituberculars (such as isoniazid, ethambutol, rifampin, and pyrazinamide) destroy or inhibit *M. tuberculosis*.
- Antibiotics (such as streptomycin) help destroy *M. tuberculosis*.

ACTIVITY

- No overexertion; alternating rest with activity

NUTRITION

- High-protein, high-carbohydrate diet
- Small, frequent meals (may be better tolerated)

loss of appetite, weight loss, intermittent fever, and fatigue. Later signs and symptoms reflect damage to other areas and may include renal failure, meningitis, and bone or joint destruction.

Health care workers, who are regularly exposed to TB, need to understand the risks and take appropriate precautions, receive regular TB testing, and obtain follow-up care as needed.

POTENTIAL COMPLICATIONS
- Lung collapse
- Pulmonary artery rupture
- Pneumothorax
- Sepsis
- Pericarditis
- Meningitis
- Renal failure
- Bone or joint destruction

TREATMENTS
- Chest percussion and drainage

RISK FACTORS
- Crowded, unsanitary, poorly ventilated living conditions
- Gender (higher incidence in men)
- Race (higher incidence in blacks and Hispanics)
- Recent immigration from Africa, Asia, Mexico, or South America
- Immunosuppression and compromised immunity
- Malnutrition
- Debilitation

AFTERCARE
- Tell the patient:
  – of the need for lifelong follow-up care
  – to avoid close contact with others until he is no longer infectious
  – that rifampin will turn body fluids orange-red
  – that family and close friends should have TB tests
  – to tell health professionals that he has TB so they can take precautions.
- Tell the patient to seek help if he has blood in sputum, difficulty breathing, increased coughing, chest pain, fever, or night sweats.

ANAPHYLAXIS

Anaphylaxis is a potentially life-threatening allergic reaction that rapidly affects several major body systems almost simultaneously. Anaphylactic reactions to drugs, insect bites, blood and blood products, and certain foods account for over 500 deaths a year in the United States. The reaction doesn't occur at the first exposure to an antigen because the body hasn't yet developed antibodies to the antigen. However, this first exposure sensitizes the body, causing it to develop antibodies that attack the antigen at subsequent exposures and trigger the reaction.

The drugs usually at fault are penicillin, iodine, and sulfonamides. Venom from bees, wasps, hornets, yellow jackets, spiders, or jellyfish can also trigger a reaction. Foods most likely to cause a reaction include shellfish, nuts, milk, strawberries, and eggs. Other allergens include yellow dye #5 and latex.

TEACHING TOPICS

MEDICATIONS

- The bronchodilator epinephrine opens the airway, raises blood pressure, and counteracts the release of histamine (available in emergency anaphylactic kits for patient use).

ACTIVITY

- Planning activities to avoid known allergens
- For activities that may expose patient to allergen, availability of an emergency anaphylaxis kit that patient and family know how to use

NUTRITION

- No known allergens or related foods; patient must check food labels
- Possible use of elimination diet to identify allergens

The anaphylactic reaction usually occurs within 30 minutes of exposure but can occur anywhere from seconds after the exposure up to an hour later. The patient feels uneasy and may become disoriented and weak. The skin—especially of the hands, feet, and genitals—becomes red and swollen, and pale, itchy wheals erupt. The patient usually feels hot and sweaty and may have vomiting and diarrhea. Initial sneezing, wheezing, and a runny nose can quickly progress to laryngospasm, bronchospasm, and asphyxia.

POTENTIAL COMPLICATIONS
- Asphyxiation
- Shock
- Cardiac or respiratory arrest

TREATMENTS
- Injection with epinephrine
- Lying still to slow circulation of the venom through the body, with an ice pack on the site of the sting
- Maintenance of a patent airway

RISK FACTORS
- Previous episode of anaphylaxis
- Asthma

AFTERCARE
- Tell the patient to:
  – keep an emergency anaphylaxis kit on hand, replace it before the expiration date, and make sure he and family or friends know how to use it
  – tell all health care professionals about all allergies so that the allergies can be documented
  – wear medical identification.
- Encourage the patient's family to take a CPR course (if appropriate).
- Tell the patient to seek help if the following occur:
  – signs and symptoms of an anaphylactic response
  – poor response to emergency anaphylaxis kit.

HEMOPHILIA

Hemophilia is a hereditary blood coagulation disorder, the main feature of which is prolonged bleeding. Before the discovery of the antihemophilic (clotting) factors, over half of hemophiliacs died in early childhood. More recently, life expectancy is near normal, unless the patient becomes sensitized to the clotting factor and develops inhibitors.

Three types of hemophilia exist: hemophilia A, hemophilia B, and von Willebrand's disease. Also called classic hemophilia, hemophilia A results from a factor VIII deficiency. It is transmitted as an X-linked, recessive trait and occurs almost exclusively in males; females are generally asymptomatic carriers. Occasionally, a genetic mutation results in hemophilia in a male with no family history of the disorder. Hemophilia B, also called Christmas disease, is a factor IX deficiency and is also transmitted as an X-linked, recessive trait. Von Willebrand's disease is a

TEACHING TOPICS

MEDICATIONS

- Clotting factor replacements (such as cryoprecipitate, lyophilized factor VIII, fresh frozen plasma, and anti-inhibitor clotting complex) supply the missing clotting factor and allow clot formation, stopping bleeding.
- Pituitary hormones with antihemorrhagic effects (such as desmopressin acetate) promote clot formation.
- Fibrinolysis inhibitors (such as aminocaproic acid) enhance clot formation.

ACTIVITY

- Regular aerobic exercise
- No contact sports (football, boxing)
- If joint problems, no activities that stress the joints (skiing, ice hockey, soccer)
- Attempt to lead as normal a life as possible

NUTRITION

- Healthy diet based on recommended portions from the food pyramid
- High-fiber diet to prevent constipation (hard, dry stools contribute to rectal tearing and hemorrhoids, which may bleed)

defect in the gene for von Willebrand factor and is transmitted as an autosomal dominant trait; it occurs in both sexes.

In severe hemophilia, the patient has a clotting factor level below 1% of the normal value; the disorder becomes apparent soon after birth, typically when a male child is circumcised. The patient with mild hemophilia may not be diagnosed until adulthood. Easy bruising, persistent or delayed bleeding after minor injuries or dental work, or joint pain and swelling may lead to the diagnosis of mild or moderate hemophilia.

Hemophilia can cause hemarthrosis, or bleeding into the joints. The recurrence of such bleeding can result in crippling joint deformities.

POTENTIAL COMPLICATIONS
- Hemorrhagic shock
- Intracranial hemorrhage

TREATMENTS
- For external bleeding, application of cold compresses and direct pressure, elevation of injured area, application of fibrin foam and topical thrombin, and visit to the doctor or emergency department
- Home infusion of clotting factor, either in response to an injury or as a prophylactic before surgery or dental work

RISK FACTORS
- Family history of hemophilia
- Gender (hemophilia A and B occur almost exclusively in males)

AFTERCARE
- Offer the patient and family emotional support and (if needed) suggest counseling.
- Tell the patient to:
  – notify all dentists and doctors about his disorder so that they can take appropriate steps
  – use an electric razor and soft toothbrush
  – wear medical identification
  – avoid aspirin and other salicylates and ibuprofen.
- Tell the patient to seek help if the following occur:
  – bleeding not responsive to clotting factor
  – symptoms of anaphylaxis.

HUMAN IMMUNODEFICIENCY VIRUS INFECTION

Human immunodeficiency virus (HIV) is a retrovirus that causes a progressive decrease in cellular immune function that leaves the patient susceptible to opportunistic infections, diseases, and cancers. HIV now affects several groups, including homosexual and bisexual men, I.V. drug users, newborns of HIV-infected women, and recipients of contaminated blood or blood products.

HIV spreads through body fluids, especially blood, semen, and vaginal secretions. Engaging in behaviors that include sharing body fluids, such as unprotected sexual contact or I.V. drug use, greatly increases the risk of contracting the virus. Nonspecific signs and symptoms—including tiredness, weight loss, after-

TEACHING TOPICS

MEDICATIONS

- Antiretrovirals (such as zidovudine, didanosine, zalcitabine, stavudine, lamivudine, saquinavir, indinavir, ritonavir, nelfinavir, nevirapine, and delavirdine) intervene at various stages of the life cycle of the virus, slowing or stalling progression of the infection.
- Drug therapies appropriate for specific complications of HIV infection treat those complications.

ACTIVITY

- Alternating activity with rest; no overexertion
- Regular aerobic exercise

NUTRITION

- High-protein, high-calorie diet
- Small, frequent meals (may be better tolerated)
- Adequate hydration
- Vitamin supplements

noon fevers, night sweats, lymph node swelling, and skin disorders—may not appear for 10 years or more after the initial infection. Complications that can affect HIV-positive patients can also occur soon after exposure.

POTENTIAL COMPLICATIONS
- *Pneumocystis carinii* pneumonia
- *Mycobacterium avium* complex
- *Cryptococcus neoformans*, candidiasis, and other fungal infections
- Cytomegalovirus retinitis
- Kaposi's sarcoma
- Malignant lymphoma
- HIV encephalopathy

TREATMENTS
- Prescribed drug regimen to control progression of HIV infection
- Specific treatments for opportunistic infections

RISK FACTORS
- Engaging in high-risk behaviors (I.V. drug use, needle or syringe sharing, unprotected sex, sex with multiple partners)
- Being born to an HIV-positive mother
- Breast-feeding from an HIV-positive woman
- Transfusion with infected blood or blood products

AFTERCARE
- Offer emotional support, and provide information about counseling and legal, financial, and community resources.
- Tell the patient to:
  – follow transmission precautions at home
  – tell all health care personnel of his HIV-positive status so they can take precautions
  – tell potential sex partners of his infection and practice safer sex
  – tell previous sex partners and anyone he shared a needle with to be tested and receive treatment.
- Tell the patient to seek help if he has a fever, difficulty breathing, a stiff neck, skin lesions, or vision changes.

RHEUMATOID ARTHRITIS

Although the cause of this chronic inflammatory disease isn't known, it's thought that the body develops altered immunoglobulin G (IgG) antibodies when exposed to an antigen. The body doesn't recognize these IgG antibodies as its own, which triggers an immune response. This results in inflammation and thickening of the synovial membranes, which can lead to breakdown of the bone and cartilage adjacent to the membranes, contractures, and joint deformities. The result can be a crippling loss of function.

Some patients have mild, easily treated symptoms; in a few, the disease progresses rapidly and quickly becomes disabling. In most patients, the disease progresses over many years, eventually becoming disabling.

TEACHING TOPICS

MEDICATIONS

- Nonsteroidal anti-inflammatory drugs (NSAIDs) decrease inflammation in joints and provide pain relief.
- Antiulcer agents help prevent gastric ulcers from NSAID use.
- Disease-modifying antirheumatic drugs reduce the autoimmune response and slow progression of the disease.
- Steroids provide short-term relief of acute inflammation and swelling.
- Hormonal agents protect against osteoporosis in women.

ACTIVITY

- No overexertion; alternating rest and exercise, pacing activities, and avoiding activities that bring on symptoms
- Using energy-efficient and joint-protection techniques and devices, with possible occupational therapy consult
- Range-of-motion and muscle-strengthening exercises and maintaining good body mechanics, with possible physical therapy consult
- Hot showers or baths (to relieve morning stiffness)

NUTRITION

- Healthy, low-fat diet based on recommended portions from the food pyramid
- No alcohol if taking NSAIDs (to lessen GI effects)
- Calcium and vitamin D supplements (to offset osteoporotic effects of corticosteroids)

No cure exists, but new drugs and drug combinations can control pain and inflammation and slow the progression of the disease. When deformities limit function, surgical resection and realignment and joint replacement may ease pain and improve mobility. Hip, knee, shoulder, and wrist replacements have met with more success than elbow and ankle replacements.

POTENTIAL COMPLICATIONS
- Active inflammation of one or more joints
- Adverse drug reactions

TREATMENTS
- Achieving and maintaining appropriate weight (to lessen strain on knees and feet)
- Hot or cold packs (for increased mobility and pain relief)
- Splints for joints as needed

RISK FACTORS
- Gender (higher incidence in women)
- Viral infections (possible; may trigger autoimmune response)
- Family history of disorder

AFTERCARE
- Tell the patient to:
  – dress warmly (cold can exacerbate stiffness and discomfort)
  – avoid over-the-counter medications without the doctor's approval
  – tell dentists and doctors about any joint replacement so prophylactic antibiotics are given before treatment.
- If the patient is worried about sexual ability, discuss pain medications, comfort measures, and alternative positions.
- Tell the patient to seek help if the following occur:
  – worsening pain
  – joint swelling or worsening of swelling
  – adverse effects that exceed the parameters set by the doctor.

SICKLE CELL SYNDROME

Sickle cell syndrome includes the genetic disorders sickle cell trait and sickle cell anemia and affects primarily blacks. A person will have sickle cell anemia if he receives the abnormal hemoglobin S (rather than the normal hemoglobin A) from both parents. He'll have sickle cell trait—a milder, sometimes asymptomatic form of the disease—if he receives the abnormal hemoglobin from only one parent. Patients with sickle cell anemia live longer than they used to but still rarely live past age 50.

In sickle cell anemia, red blood cells contain the abnormal hemoglobin. These cells have a normal oxygen-carrying ability but become hard and sickle shaped when oxygen levels in the blood decrease. Conditions that increase the body's need for oxygen—such as high altitudes, unusually strenuous exercise, pregnancy, and anesthesia—can result in a painful vaso-occlusive crisis in which

TEACHING TOPICS

MEDICATIONS

- Folic acid supplements (such as vitamin B_9) stimulate blood cell and platelet production.
- Analgesics (such as acetaminophen) or narcotic analgesics (during painful crises) lessen pain.
- Antibiotics (such as low-dose oral penicillin) prevent infection.

ACTIVITY

- Regular activity as tolerated while maintaining hydration; no overexertion
- No contact sports for patient with splenomegaly

NUTRITION

- Foods high in folic acid
- Adequate hydration (especially important)

the red blood cells sickle, clump together, and thicken the blood. Dehydration—from sweating, vomiting, or diarrhea—worsens the patient's condition. If normal oxygenation and hydration aren't restored, infarction and possibly necrosis may occur.

POTENTIAL COMPLICATIONS
- Vaso-occlusive crisis
- Cerebral hemorrhage
- Renal failure, shock
- Respiratory failure, pneumonia
- Myocardial infarction
- Sepsis
- Osteomyelitis
- Cholelithiasis

TREATMENTS
- Smoking cessation and avoiding second-hand smoke
- Oxygen therapy
- Pneumococcal and influenza virus (including hemophilus influenza type B) vaccinations

RISK FACTORS
- Race (occurs mainly in blacks and in those who live in tropical Africa or the Mediterranean region)

AFTERCARE
- Offer the patient and family emotional support and (if needed) suggest counseling.
- Tell the patient to:
  – receive genetic counseling before marriage and childbearing
  – notify all health care professionals of his disorder
  – consider wearing medical identification.
- Tell the patient to seek help if he has difficulty breathing, fever, vomiting, diarrhea, stiff neck, joint or abdominal pain, difficulty walking or talking, dizziness, or jaundice.

SYSTEMIC LUPUS ERYTHEMATOSUS

Systemic lupus erythematosus is an autoimmune disorder in which the body produces antibodies to its own antigens and forms immune complexes that cause inflammation and possible damage to most major body systems. Signs and symptoms of this chronic disorder can range from mild to potentially fatal, and progression of the disorder can vary greatly. Patients typically experience periods of remission that are irregularly interrupted by exacerbations.

Signs and symptoms include photosensitive rashes (including facial erythema), joint stiffness and pain, and fever and unusual tiredness. Pleuritic chest pain and difficulty breathing can also occur. Stress, infections, and exposure to sunlight may bring on exacerbations.

TEACHING TOPICS

MEDICATIONS

- Sunscreens with at least SPF 15 for UVB protection and micronized titanium dioxide for UVA protection guard against photosensitivity.
- NSAIDs decrease joint inflammation and relieve pain.
- Steroids relieve inflammation and skin lesions.
- Antimalarials promote healing of skin lesions.
- Immunosuppressants may sometimes be used in place of systemic steroids to avoid the adverse effects of long-term steroid use.

ACTIVITY

- Pacing activities; moderate exercise alternating with rest; exercise should stop if fatigue occurs
- Adequate sleep at night (around 10 hours) and rest periods during the day

NUTRITION

- Regular diet unless complication occurs
- Sufficient iron to prevent anemia

Treatment varies with the type and severity of the symptoms; the patient may only need protection from the sun and topical steroids and possibly nonsteroidal anti-inflammatory drugs (NSAIDs). More severe skin lesions or joint symptoms may require systemic steroids, antimalarials, or immunosuppressants.

POTENTIAL COMPLICATIONS
- Cardiac arrest
- Renal failure
- Seizures
- Psychosis
- Peripheral neuropathy, possibly with gangrene of fingers and toes

Treatments
- Hot or cold packs (to improve mobility and provide pain relief)
- Stress reduction and relaxation techniques and biofeedback
- Prompt treatment of infections

Risk Factors
- Gender (much higher incidence in women)
- Race (higher incidence in Asians and blacks)
- Age (adults ages 20 to 50)
- Family history of systemic lupus erythematosus
- Bacterial or viral infections
- Immunizations

Aftercare
- Tell the patient:
  – to stay out of sunlight, apply sunscreen frequently, and wear protective clothing when outdoors
  – that pregnancy is risky and can worsen disease
  – that oral contraceptives may be contraindicated
  – to receive eye examinations for retinal changes
  –to receive pneumonia and flu shots.
- Tell patient to seek help if any of the following occur:
  – fever
  – cough
  – skin rash
  – worsening chest, abdominal, muscle, or joint pain
  – unusually heavy or lengthy menstrual flow.

THROMBOCYTOPENIA

In thrombocytopenia, a decrease in the number of blood platelets prevents the formation of platelet plugs at breaks in the skin, which interferes with normal clot formation and healing. This drop in the number of platelets may result from fewer platelets being made, more platelets being destroyed, or platelets being abnormally distributed. Thrombocytopenia can be a primary immune disorder or induced by drugs or alcohol; it may also result from another disease, viral infection, or vitamin deficiency.

A patient who has no symptoms may only have the disorder detected during blood tests for another reason. Most patients have nasal, GI, or genitourinary bleeding or purpura (petechiae and ecchymoses) that results from red blood cells

TEACHING TOPICS

MEDICATIONS

- Steroids (such as betamethasone, cortisone, prednisolone, prednisone, and triamcinolone) lessen the immune response.
- Immunosuppressants (such as cyclosporine) decrease the immune response.

ACTIVITY

- Possibly no strenuous exercise or contact or injury-intensive sports

NUTRITION

- Healthy diet based on recommended portions from the food pyramid

leaking into the skin and mucous membranes. Hematomas may also occur from mild injuries.

Treatment for the acute phase of the disorder depends on the cause and mechanism of the thrombocytopenia and the patient's platelet count. In some instances, the patient may require splenectomy.

POTENTIAL COMPLICATIONS
- Acute hemorrhage (intracranial, GI, or intrapulmonary or cardiac tamponade)

TREATMENTS
- Humidifier (to keep nasal membranes moist and prevent bleeding)

RISK FACTORS
- Predisposing disorders (viral infections, immune disorders, tuberculosis)
- Some medicines (gold salts, procainamide, quinidine, quinine, sulfa, sulfa derivatives, valproic acid)
- Toxins (insecticides, exposure to radiation)

AFTERCARE
- Tell the patient:
  – to wear medical identification
  – how to manage Cushing's syndrome (if undergoing long-term steroid treatment)
  – to use cold compresses, fibrin foam, and topical thrombin and to apply firm pressure on any cut and keep cut elevated above heart level if possible; if bleeding continues, the patient should go to the emergency department.
- Tell the patient to seek help if the following occur:
  – bleeding from the mucous membranes or GI tract
  – increasing numbers of petechiae or ecchymoses
  – unusually heavy or lengthy menstrual flow.

ALZHEIMER'S DISEASE

Alzheimer's disease causes a progressive loss of memory, intellect, personality, and function, culminating in dementia and death. It accounts for half of all dementias and causes over 100,000 deaths each year in the United States. Although its causes aren't known, it's associated with age, heredity, the apolipoprotein E genotype, head injury, and possibly viruses and toxins. Autopsies reveal senile plaques, neurofibrillary tangles, and vascular amyloid in the brain.

Onset typically occurs after age 60, although it can occur as early as age 40. The patient initially complains of recent memory loss; he has trouble remembering names and where he placed items. As the disease progresses, the patient loses the ability to concentrate and to focus on more than one thing at a time and may

TEACHING TOPICS

MEDICATIONS

- Anticholinergics (such as tacrine and donepezil) help maintain cognitive function.
- Antidepressants (such as fluoxetine, paroxetine, sertraline, trazodone, and venlafaxine) may improve depression.
- Low doses of antianxiety agents (such as lorazepam, alprazolam, and buspirone) may relieve anxiety.
- Antipsychotics (such as haloperidol, risperidone, and thioridazine) may reduce agitation.
- Sleeping aids (such as zolpidem, diphenhydramine, and short-acting benzodiazepine [short-term use]) may relieve insomnia.

ACTIVITY

- Supervised, regular aerobic or isometric exercises for as long as possible
- Reality-orienting activities (references to clocks and calendars, verbal reminders)

NUTRITION

- High-fiber, high-calorie diet
- One course offered at a time (patient may eat more)
- Monitoring of chewing and swallowing
- Bite-size or soft foods (as disease progresses)

develop insomnia. Other signs and symptoms—typically noted by family or friends—include depression, withdrawal, delusions, hallucinations, personality changes, and atypical behaviors. Slowly, the patient loses his ability to manage self-care, speak, and comprehend. He may experience anxiety, agitation, and fearfulness and may wander off, unable to communicate or find his way home. In the final stages, the patient doesn't recognize himself or others and becomes incontinent and physically disabled. By this point, home care usually becomes unmanageable. Death typically occurs from 6 to 10 years after onset of the disease.

POTENTIAL COMPLICATIONS
- Aspiration pneumonia
- Injury (such as burns)

TREATMENTS

- Incontinence management (adult diapers, pads, bedside commode)
- Psychiatric, social, and geriatric consults may be needed

RISK FACTORS

- Family history of Alzheimer's disease
- Age (adults over age 60)
- Apolipoprotein E genotype
- Gender (higher incidence in women)
- Head injury

AFTERCARE

- Offer the patient and family support, particularly the primary caregiver
- Tell the caregiver to:
  – maintain a regular, relatively unchanging schedule in familiar surroundings
  – lock away medicines, toxins, and dangerous items as needed
  – have the patient taking tacrine receive liver function monitoring, as ordered
  – make sure the patient wears medical identification.
- Tell the caregiver to seek help if:
  – the patient has fever, difficulty breathing, or behaves dangerously
  – the caregiver is unable to cope.

AMYOTROPHIC LATERAL SCLEROSIS

Also called Lou Gehrig's disease, amyotrophic lateral sclerosis progressively robs the patient of movement while leaving sensory and intellectual abilities intact. The cause of the disease is unknown, but degeneration of upper and lower motor neurons leads to muscle weakness and wasting. Most patients die within 3 years of onset, usually from aspiration, infection, or respiratory failure.

The disease typically affects the muscles of the hands first, resulting in loss of fine motor skills and clumsiness. Impaired speech and difficulty swallowing and breathing follow. Muscle wasting progresses downward, affecting the legs and feet last, although most patients maintain bowel and bladder control until close to the

TEACHING TOPICS

MEDICATIONS

- Glutamate antagonists (such as riluzole) slow the progression of the disease.
- Skeletal muscle relaxants (such as baclofen and dantrolene) ease muscle spasms.
- Antidepressants (such as amitriptyline, fluoxetine, nefazodone, paroxetine, sertraline, and venlafaxine) help manage depression.

ACTIVITY

- Stretching, range-of-motion, and strengthening exercises
- Energy-conservation measures and equipment, with possible occupational therapy consult
- Using walker or wheelchair as needed, with possible physical therapy consult

NUTRITION

- High-calorie, high-fiber, high-protein diet
- Eating in upright position and chewing food thoroughly
- Bite-size or soft foods as needed
- Small, frequent meals (may provide better nutrition)
- No sticky, mucus-producing foods (peanut butter, milk)
- Nasogastric or gastrostomy tube feedings as needed (to avoid aspiration)

end. Other signs and symptoms include atrophy, cramping, spasms, and hyper-reflexia of the muscles as well as fatigue and depression.

Riluzole slows the progression of the disease. Otherwise, treatment aims to control symptoms and maintain the patient's physical and emotional comfort.

POTENTIAL COMPLICATIONS
- Respiratory infection
- Respiratory failure
- Aspiration
- Atelectasis
- Injuries from falling
- Infection (of pressure ulcer)
- Sepsis

TREATMENTS
- Oxygen therapy
- Suctioning (as need-ed)
- Deep-breathing exer-cises
- Skin care program to prevent pressure ul-cers (turning, mas-sage, elbow and heel covers, sheepskin, convoluted foam or air mattress, foot-board)
- Mechanical ventila-tion (may be needed as disease progresses)

RISK FACTORS
- Family history of amy-otrophic lateral scle-rosis
- Location (higher inci-dence in Guam)
- Gender (higher inci-dence in men)

AFTERCARE
- Offer the patient and family support.
- If the patient needs a cervi-cal collar, brace, or splints, teach him how to use them.
- Teach caregivers to use and maintain a mechanical ven-tilator and related equip-ment.
- Tell the patient to receive pneumonia shots and flu shots, as recommended.
- Tell the patient's caregiver to seek help if the following occur:
  - inability to manage saliva
  - difficulty swallowing
  - fever
  - skin breakdown on back.

BELL'S PALSY

Also called acute peripheral facial paralysis, Bell's palsy affects the seventh cranial (facial) nerve, resulting in unilateral facial paralysis. A patient with Bell's palsy can't wrinkle his forehead, blink or close his eye, or control his lips on the affected side. When the patient tries to close his eye, it rolls upward (Bell's phenomenon) and shows excessive tearing. The patient may drool and lose the ability to chew. Taste perception may also be distorted over the affected anterior portion of the tongue.

Bell's palsy occurs in all age-groups, but is most common in people under age 60. The condition subsides spontaneously in 80% to 90% of all patients; complete recovery results within 1 to 8 weeks; however, recovery may be delayed in

TEACHING TOPICS

MEDICATIONS

- Steroids (such as prednisone) reduce inflammation and swelling.
- Antivirals (such as famciclovir and acyclovir) combat viral infection.

ACTIVITY

- Facial exercises performed several times daily in front of a mirror when motor ability starts to return

NUTRITION

- Healthy diet based on recommended portions from the food pyramid

older adults. If partial recovery occurs, contractures may develop on the paralyzed side. Bell's palsy may recur on the same or opposite side of the face.

Bell's palsy appears to be an inflammatory response to a herpes simplex infection; it can also follow facial trauma or a stroke. It usually comes on suddenly and peaks in about 2 weeks. Treatment includes eye protection and medication; some patients may need surgery.

POTENTIAL COMPLICATIONS
- Corneal irritation or damage

TREATMENTS
- Gentle massage of the affected side
- Moist heat applied to the affected side
- Electrical stimulation of the affected facial nerve
- Eye patch and eye-drops or ointment for the affected eye

RISK FACTORS
- Viral infections
- Facial trauma
- Stroke

AFTERCARE
- Tell the patient to wear sunglasses when outdoors.
- Offer the patient emotional support.
- Tell the patient to seek help if he experiences redness, irritation, or drainage from the eye.

CEREBROVASCULAR ACCIDENT

Commonly called a stroke, cerebrovascular accident (CVA) is the leading cause of severe disability and the third leading cause of death in the United States. However, the incidence of CVA is declining, possibly because of better treatments for cardiovascular disease.

In CVA, ischemia or hemorrhage within the brain results in neurologic damage. Ischemia accounts for about 90% of CVAs, and the CVA itself may be preceded by transient ischemic attacks. Thrombus formation within the brain secondary to atherosclerosis accounts for most ischemic CVAs, although emboli from the heart, arteries, or veins can also trigger an ischemic CVA. Improved management of hypertension has reduced the incidence of hemorrhagic CVA to about 10%. Besides hypertension, causes of hemorrhagic CVA include aneurysms, arteriovenous malformation, and abuse of certain drugs (such as amphetamines and cocaine).

The main sign of CVA is hemiparesis; the patient may also have vision changes or lose sensation and the ability to talk. The full extent of neurologic

TEACHING TOPICS

MEDICATIONS

- Antihypertensives maintain normal blood pressure.
- Antiplatelets slow blood clotting, helping to prevent clot formation.
- Platelet aggregation inhibitors prevent platelets from clumping, helping to reduce thrombus formation.
- Hemorrheologics reduce blood viscosity, helping to prevent thrombus formation.
- Anticoagulants help prevent clot formation.
- Antidepressants combat depression.

ACTIVITY

- Range-of-motion, strengthening, and ambulation exercises
- Use of adaptive techniques and devices for activities of daily living
- Speech, comprehension, and swallowing therapy
- Continuing exercise program as able after discharge
- Turning

NUTRITION

- Low-salt diet for hypertensive patient
- Possible low-fat diet
- Adequate hydration
- Achieving and maintaining appropriate weight
- Soft foods as needed

damage occurs quickly, typically within an hour, and almost a quarter of acute CVA patients die during the initial hospitalization. Administration of tissue plasminogen activator within the first few hours of the CVA has been shown to minimize damage by dissolving the thrombus.

Rehabilitation for those who survive starts almost immediately after the acute phase in an attempt to minimize the impact of the CVA and maximize the patient's ability to function. The patient and family need education, psychological support and counseling, and referrals to financial and community resources.

POTENTIAL COMPLICATIONS
- Increased intracranial pressure
- Herniation
- Aspiration pneumonia
- Seizures
- Deep vein thrombosis and embolus

TREATMENTS
- Stress management and relaxation techniques and biofeedback.
- Splinting of limbs as necessary (to prevent contractures)
- Smoking cessation
- Coughing and deep breathing as needed (to maintain respiratory function)

RISK FACTORS
- Age (adults ages 50 to 80)
- Atherosclerosis
- Heart disease
- Hypertension
- Diabetes mellitus
- Obesity
- Abuse of amphetamines and cocaine

AFTERCARE
- Remind the family to allow the patient to do as much as possible without help or he won't maintain abilities he recovered during therapy.
- Discuss the availability of day rehabilitation facilities.
- Tell the patient to seek help if the following occur:
  – headache, dizziness, vision changes
  – confusion
  – seizures
  – difficulty breathing
  – worsening of functional abilities.

HEADACHES

Headaches can be classified as vascular, tension, or traction and inflammatory. Vascular headaches include migraine, cluster, facial, toxic, and hypertensive headaches.

Migraines, the most common type of vascular headache, affect mostly women, often in relation to the menstrual cycle. Some patients experience an aura before a migraine headache starts.

Cluster headaches can last from a few minutes to about 4 hours and are accompanied by ptosis, tearing, flushing, and sweating. They characteristically happen in series that last from 1 to 3 months during which time the patient may have several headaches a day. After that, the patient has a headache-free period that can last for years.

TEACHING TOPICS

MEDICATIONS

- To prevent migraine: calcium channel blockers, tricyclic antidepressants (TCAs), anticonvulsants, beta blockers, adrenergic blockers, and serotonin selective agonists
- To relieve severe migraine: narcotic analgesics
- To stop migraines: nonsteroidal anti-inflammatory drugs (NSAIDs)
- To prevent cluster headaches: antimanics, calcium channel blockers, and NSAIDs
- To reduce cluster headache pain and inflammation: steroids
- To stop cluster headaches: adrenergic blockers and serotonin selective agonists
- To prevent tension headaches: TCAs and antidepressants
- To stop tension headaches: NSAIDs

ACTIVITY

- Regular aerobic exercise (helps prevent tension and possibly migraine headaches)
- For migraine patients, avoiding or adapting to known triggers (fatigue, changes in weather or altitude, going too long without food, bright lights, certain odors, onset of menstrual cycle, oversleeping)
- Keeping a headache history (to recognize patterns, triggers, and correlations that may help in headache management)

NUTRITION

- No tyramine-rich foods (aged cheese and chocolate; alcohol; caffeine; dried, fermented, smoked, or pickled foods; flavorings such as monosodium glutamate) if they trigger migraine headaches
- Eating regularly (may help prevent migraine headaches)
- No nitrates (in foods such as cured meats and drugs such as nitroglycerin) for cluster headache patients

Tension headaches generally begin slowly, without throbbing, and cause pain and tightness in the neck. Some patients have mixed headache syndrome, experiencing both tension and migraine headaches.

Indications that a headache signals a more serious disorder include:
- a description of the headache as "the worst headache of my life"
- onset of headaches after age 45
- onset of a type of headache the patient doesn't usually experience
- headache accompanied by a change in consciousness, weakness, tingling, numbness, loss of hearing, vision changes, fever, or sore or pulsating temporal arteries.

POTENTIAL COMPLICATIONS
- Blindness if headache results from temporal arteritis

Treatments

- Smoking cessation
- Lying down in a dark, quiet room with cold compresses to the head (may relax and relieve pain of migraine or tension headache)
- Stress management and relaxation techniques and biofeedback (for some types of vascular and tension headaches)

Risk factors

- Family history of migraine headaches
- Gender (higher incidence in women, especially of migraines; higher incidence of cluster headaches in men)

Aftercare

- Teach the patient how to use an aerosol (as appropriate).
- Tell the patient to seek help if the following occur:
  – migraine headache that lasts several days or weeks
  – unbearable pain
  – unusual vision changes.

MULTIPLE SCLEROSIS

Also called disseminated sclerosis, multiple sclerosis (MS) is a central nervous system disease that results in scattered areas of demyelination of nerves, which lead to patches of sclerotic tissue. Chronic, progressive, and usually degenerative, MS is characterized by periods of remission and exacerbation. What causes the destruction of the myelin sheath isn't known, but viral infection is a possibility.

The disease usually affects young adults and occurs in two basic forms. Most patients have a pattern of relapse and remission, with remission most likely stemming from healing of demyelinated sites. As the disease progresses, however, degeneration of nerve fibers becomes irreversible. A few patients have primary chronic progressive MS, which results in severe disability in a very few years.

TEACHING TOPICS

MEDICATIONS

- Antiviral, immunoregulators protect cells from viral infection.
- Antivirals reduce relapse severity and frequency.
- Biological response modifiers decrease the frequency of attacks and the severity of disability.
- Immunosuppressants slow disease progression in some patients.
- Antidepressants help manage depression.
- Anticholinergics relieve urinary urgency.
- Skeletal muscle relaxants ease muscle spasms.
- Steroids reduce inflammation and swelling during acute attacks.
- Surfactant laxatives help manage chronic constipation.

ACTIVITY

- Planning activities around peak energy periods, and alternating activity with rest to prevent overexertion
- Gentle stretching, range-of-motion, and strengthening exercises, with possible physical therapy consult
- Recognizing and managing stressors
- Possible gait retraining or use of a cane, walker, or wheelchair
- If sensory loss, watching arms and legs regularly to prevent injury

NUTRITION

- High-fiber diet (to relieve constipation)
- Adequate fluid intake (to prevent constipation and urinary infections)
- Cranberry or other acidic juices (to combat bladder infection)
- Soft foods (during periods of exacerbation)
- Eating slowly (to prevent aspiration)
- Possible high-calorie diet (if patient can't eat much)

Signs and symptoms of MS vary greatly, depending on where demyelination occurs. Many patients suffer fatigue, depression, and sexual dysfunction. Sensory symptoms can include some degree of loss of feeling, burning or tingling, and pain. Motor signs and symptoms can include partial or complete paralysis, muscle spasms, foot dragging, double vision, and either incontinence or bowel or bladder retention. Patients may also experience loss of muscle coordination, loss of balance, speaking difficulties, dizziness, and tremors.

POTENTIAL COMPLICATIONS
- Respiratory failure
- Paralysis
- Injury from falls
- Urinary tract infections

TREATMENTS
- Stress management techniques
- Bowel and bladder retraining (as needed)
- Self-catheterization or Credé's method (to empty bladder)

RISK FACTORS
- Gender (higher incidence in women)
- Race (higher incidence in whites)
- Age (adults ages 30 to 50)
- Location (higher incidence in northern, colder climates)
- Family history of MS
- Viral infections (possible trigger)

AFTERCARE
- Offer emotional support, suggest counseling as needed, and expect emotional lability (which may be partly organic).
- Arrange for sexual counseling as needed (MS typically causes sexual dysfunction).
- Arrange for speech therapy as needed.
- Tell the patient:
  – to avoid crowds and people with infections
  – to wear medical identification
  – that pregnancy may make symptoms worse.
- Tell the patient to seek help if the following occur:
  – urinary tract infection
  – fever
  – confusion or disorientation.

MYASTHENIA GRAVIS

In myasthenia gravis, reduced numbers of acetylcholine receptors on muscles and larger-than-normal gaps at neuromuscular junctions prevent normal transmission of nerve impulses to muscles, resulting in muscle weakness. This chronic disease is thought to result from an autoimmune response that triggers the production of acetylcholine receptor antibodies. Myasthenia gravis is also linked with other autoimmune diseases, such as rheumatoid arthritis and systemic lupus erythematosus.

The rate of onset and degree of muscle weakness vary greatly, and periods of remission and exacerbation generally occur. Exacerbation can result from infection, stress, hormones, and certain drugs. Symptoms of the disease begin with weakness that first appears in face muscles (drooping eyelids and double vision)

TEACHING TOPICS

MEDICATIONS

- Anticholinesterase agents (such as pyridostigmine bromide and ephedrine) prevent acetylcholine breakdown and improve transmission of nerve impulses.
- Steroids (such as prednisone) suppress inflammation from the autoimmune reaction.
- Immunosuppressants (such as azathioprine and cyclosporine) reduce the autoimmune response.
- Antidiarrheals (such as atropine sulfate and loperamide hydrochloride) prevent diarrhea that can result from anticholinesterase agents.

ACTIVITY

- Planning activities around peak energy periods, and alternating activity with rest to prevent overexertion
- Planning medication so that peak effects coincide with meals and activities
- Energy-conservation measures and equipment, with possible occupational therapy consult
- Recognizing and managing stressors

NUTRITION

- Soft foods and liquids mixed with foods to prevent aspiration (during periods of exacerbation)
- Eating slowly (to prevent aspiration)
- Possible high-calorie diet (if patient can't eat much)

and progresses downward. The patient may have trouble holding his head up and raising his arms, and his fingers may grow weak. His speech may become nasal and whispery, and he may have trouble swallowing. When the disease affects respiratory muscles, the patient may experience a myasthenic crisis and require mechanical ventilation. As the disease progresses downward, the patient may lose bowel and bladder control and function and the ability to walk.

POTENTIAL COMPLICATIONS
- Myasthenic crisis
- Cholinergic crisis
- Respiratory failure
- Aspiration pneumonia

TREATMENTS
- No alcohol (exacerbates the muscle weakness)
- Handheld resuscitation bag and suctioning available at home (for patient at risk for respiratory crises)
- Eyedrops and eye protection, possibly with eye patch (for severe ptosis)
- Surgical removal of thymus, as appropriate, to support immune system

RISK FACTORS
- Treatment with D-penicillamine (given for rheumatoid arthritis or Wilson's disease)
- Gender and age (higher incidence in adolescent and young women females and in males ages 50 to 60)

AFTERCARE
- Tell the female patient:
  – that symptoms may grow better or worse during pregnancy or may not change at all
  – that any offspring should be checked for neonatal myasthenia gravis.
- Tell the patient to:
  – pay close attention to respiratory symptoms if he has asthma
  – receive pneumonia vaccinations every 10 years and yearly flu vaccinations; although unlikely, symptoms may worsen after flu vaccination
  – wear medical identification.
- Tell the patient to seek help if he has difficulty breathing, increasing weakness, fever, more difficulty than usual speaking, or an infection.

PARKINSON'S DISEASE

A progressive disorder, Parkinson's disease causes deterioration and debilitation from involuntary tremor, slowed ability to initiate movement, muscle rigidity, loss of postural reflexes, and the freezing phenomenon. Death usually occurs about 10 years after onset.

The motor changes characteristic of Parkinson's disease result from a gradual loss of dopamine-containing neurons in the brain, which causes a drop in dopamine levels. The disease is classified by etiology. The cause of primary Parkinson's disease is unknown. Secondary parkinsonism may result from drugs, viruses, or toxins. Parkinsonism-plus syndromes include palsies and dementias, and heredodegenerative diseases include such conditions as juvenile Huntington's disease.

Other characteristic features of Parkinson's disease besides motor degeneration include depression, confusion, agitation, constipation, excessive sleeping, delusions, hallucinations, and psychosis, although some of these signs and symptoms may result from the drugs taken to treat the disorder.

TEACHING TOPICS

MEDICATIONS

- Antiparkinsonian agents (such as selegiline, levodopa, pergolide, and bromocriptine) lessen motor symptoms.
- Antivirals (such as amantadine) promote release of dopamine in the brain, helping to relieve motor symptoms.
- Anticholinergic drugs (such as trihexyphenidyl and benztropine mesylate) decrease tremors.
- Antidepressants (such as amitriptyline, protriptyline, nefazodone, and venlafaxine) help treat depression.
- Bulk-forming laxatives (such as methylcellulose and psyllium) help relieve constipation.

ACTIVITY

- Regular aerobic exercise, alternating activity with rest
- Energy-conservation measures and equipment as needed, with possible occupational therapy consult

NUTRITION

- Monitoring of chewing and swallowing
- High-fiber, high-calorie diet
- Possible decreased protein diet
- Adequate hydration
- Bite-size food as needed

Although levodopa is the main drug used to treat Parkinson's disease, complications can arise from long-term use. Because of this, the patient may be advised to use other drugs first and wait until the disease reaches a moderate level before starting levodopa therapy. At that point, he should receive the lowest effective dose, usually in combination with other drugs. He then receives increasing doses of levodopa as needed to control symptoms until complications from the drug outweigh its benefits. Depression, which is common in Parkinson's disease, can prevent the maximum benefit of antiparkinsonian drugs, so the patient may also receive antidepressants and possibly electroconvulsive therapy.

Alternative treatments for Parkinson's disease are being tried on some patients, and the development of new drugs and therapies continues. Experimental surgical procedures include thalamotomy, pallidotomy, deep brain stimulation, and fetal tissue implantation.

POTENTIAL COMPLICATIONS
- Aspiration pneumonia
- Dementia

TREATMENTS

- Stress management and relaxation techniques
- Splints or braces as needed
- Physical and speech therapy, as needed
- Surgical measures, such as adrenal medullary transplants, thalamotomy, stereotaxic pallidotomy, or deep brain stimulation, as appropriate

RISK FACTORS

- Age (adults over age 60)
- Certain drugs (dopamine receptor blockers, dopamine storage depletors)
- Toxins (manganese, carbon monoxide, cyanide)
- Certain disorders (palsies, Shy-Drager syndrome, dementias, Wilson's disease, juvenile Huntington's disease)

AFTERCARE

- Offer the patient and family support, and arrange for social and psychological services as needed.
- Provide opportunities for socialization and intellectual stimulation.
- Tell the patient that he shouldn't stop taking levodopa suddenly because this may bring on neuroleptic malignant syndrome.
- Tell the patient or caregiver to seek help if the following occur:
  – fever
  – difficulty breathing
  – decreasing effectiveness of drugs
  – inability of caregiver to cope.

SEIZURE DISORDER

Also called epilepsy, seizure disorder is a condition of the brain marked by a susceptibility to recurrent seizures. In most cases, the cause is unknown. About 20% of patients initially diagnosed with seizure disorder actually have other conditions, including syncope, drug-induced seizures, and psychological disorders.

An epileptic seizure can be categorized as partial or generalized. In a partial seizure, the patient may or may not lose consciousness. Several types of generalized seizures can occur, but the most common type is the generalized tonic-clonic seizure. In this type of seizure, the patient's level of consciousness changes, and his movements are bilateral. Before the seizure, the patient may experience a prodromal period when he feels irritable and tense. This period can last for up to a few days. Just before a seizure, the patient may experience an aura, although some patients have no warning. During the first, or tonic, phase of the seizure, the patient's voluntary muscles contract. He may cry out and fall to the ground,

TEACHING TOPICS

MEDICATIONS

- Anticonvulsants (such as carbamazepine, clonazepam, ethosuximide, felbamate, gabapentin, lamotrigine, phenobarbital, phenytoin, primidone, valproic acid, and divalproex) prevent or reduce excessive neuron discharge, preventing or decreasing the frequency of seizures.

ACTIVITY

- Avoiding or adapting to known triggers (fatigue, insufficient sleep, going too long without food, bright lights, certain odors, certain types of music, emotional stress, electric shock, fever, constipation, hyperventilation, onset of menstrual cycle)
- Keeping a seizure and medication calendar (to recognize patterns, triggers, and correlations that may help in seizure management)

NUTRITION

- Supplemental B-complex vitamins and folic acid (to offset dietary effects of anticonvulsants)

bite his tongue, lose bowel and bladder control, and stop breathing. This phase usually lasts less than a minute. The clonic phase, which usually lasts about 30 seconds, follows. In this phase, the patient has jerky, regular muscle contractions and hyperventilates. He may also salivate and froth at the mouth, contort his face, roll his eyes back in his head, and sweat. After the seizure, the patient's muscles relax and his pupils begin to respond, although he may remain unconscious for up to 5 minutes. If seizures continue for over 30 minutes without stopping or if two or more seizures occur without full recovery of consciousness between them, the patient has the life-threatening condition called status epilepticus.

POTENTIAL COMPLICATIONS
- Brain damage
- Accidental injuries
- Brain tumor

TREATMENTS
- Seizure first aid:
  – help the patient lie down (if necessary) and have a family member or other caregiver stay with him
  – remove any glasses and loosen restrictive clothing
  – don't put anything in his mouth
  – guide his movements away from anything that could injure, but don't restrain him
  – place him on his side after the seizure and orient him to time and place when he awakens.

RISK FACTORS
- Head injury
- Central nervous system infections (meningitis, encephalitis, abscesses)
- Brain tumors
- Cerebral vascular disease (strokes, arteriovenous malformations, cerebral aneurysms)

AFTERCARE
- Provide the patient and family with information about legislative issues and community resources.
- Offer emotional support (depression is common) and suggest counseling as needed to help the patient and family cope with the social stigma that commonly accompanies epilepsy.
- Tell the patient to wear medical identification.
- Explain the dangers of suddenly stopping anticonvulsants.
- Tell the patient to seek help if the following occur:
  – recurrence or worsening of seizures
  – change in type of seizure.

TRIGEMINAL NEURALGIA

Also called tic douloureux, trigeminal neuralgia is a painful, sometimes disabling disorder of one or more of the three main branches of the fifth cranial (trigeminal) nerve. The disorder usually affects the third branch of the nerve and typically affects only one side of the face. Patients with multiple sclerosis have a higher incidence of this disorder.

The largest cranial nerve, the trigeminal nerve provides motor and sensory function for much of the face, including the forehead, eyes, nose, upper and lower jaws, lips, teeth, gums, tongue, and parts of the ears. Trigeminal neuralgia is thought to result when atherosclerotic blood vessels compress the nerve at the point where it reenters the brain; demyelination may also occur at the site of compression.

Trigeminal neuralgia is characterized by periods when painful attacks can occur anywhere from several times a day to several times a month alternating with

TEACHING TOPICS

MEDICATIONS

- Anticonvulsants (such as carbamazepine, gabapentin, and phenytoin) decrease facial pain (pain relief from carbamazepine confirms the diagnosis of trigeminal neuralgia).
- Skeletal muscle relaxants (such as baclofen) lessen facial pain if the patient can't take carbamazepine or gabapentin.
- Narcotic analgesics (such as meperidine and codeine) relieve facial pain.

ACTIVITY

- Modifying activities to avoid or manage pain triggers (staying warm and out of cold winds, covering the face with a scarf when going outside)
- Regular aerobic exercise

NUTRITION

- No chewing on affected side
- Small, frequent meals (may be easier to manage)
- High-calorie diet as needed
- Soft or pureed room-temperature foods as needed during active periods (possible nutritional consult)

pain-free periods that can sometimes last from months to years. When the disorder is active, the patient typically has a sensitive zone around the mouth, on the gums and teeth, or on the forehead that responds to such triggers as touch, talking, tooth brushing, chewing, sudden temperature changes, or a blast of cold air. When this sensitive zone is triggered, it causes searing, paroxysmal pain that can last anywhere from a few seconds to a few minutes. The patient may fear triggering pain so much that he won't eat, talk, or brush his teeth, which can result in weight loss, social isolation, and dental and gingival problems. Medication can help control pain; various surgeries, some minimally invasive, can usually help when pain medication proves ineffective.

POTENTIAL COMPLICATIONS
- Malnutrition and weight loss
- Depression
- Infections or disease of the teeth and gums

TREATMENTS
- Maintaining appropriate weight
- Surgical measures, such as microvascular decompression of the fifth cranial nerve, partial sensory rhizotomy, peripheral nerve block, or peripheral nerve ablation, as appropriate

RISK FACTORS
- Gender (higher incidence in women)
- Age (adults over age 60)
- Atherosclerosis
- Facial trauma
- Oral surgery
- Multiple sclerosis

AFTERCARE
- Monitor the white blood cell count of the patient taking carbamazepine or phenytoin.
- Tell the patient to:
  – weigh himself daily, record weights, and report sudden or steady changes
  – avoid rubbing the eye on the affected side after surgery that affects sensory function.
- Tell the patient to seek help if the following occur:
  – increasing pain
  – decreasing effectiveness of prescribed medicine
  – sudden or steady weight loss
  – depression.

CHOLECYSTITIS

Cholecystitis is an acute or chronic inflammation of the gallbladder. Older, obese women have a higher incidence of this disorder.

Acute cholecystitis—also called biliary colic—typically results when the gallbladder contracts in an attempt to pass bile through a bile duct blocked by a gallstone. The main symptom is severe, sudden pain in the epigastric or subscapular areas, and the patient may experience nausea and vomiting; occasionally, fever and, rarely, jaundice also occur. Treatment options include drug treatment to dissolve the stones (possibly with methyl tert-butyl ether), lithotripsy to crush the stones, and laparoscopic or open abdominal surgery (cholecystectomy) to remove the stones.

Acute cholecystitis that doesn't result from a stone blocking a bile duct is called acalculous cholecystitis. It can result from major trauma, surgery, multiple blood transfusions, sepsis secondary to infection with gram-negative bacteria, fast-

TEACHING TOPICS

MEDICATIONS

- Anticholinergics (such as dicyclomine and glycopyrrolate) reduce spasms of the biliary tract muscle.
- Digestive enzymes and gallstone solubilizers (such as chenodiol and ursodiol) shrink or dissolve cholesterol gallstones.
- Antacids (such as magnesium-aluminum hydroxides, aluminum hydroxides, and calcium carbonates) inhibit gastric acid secretion and provide relief from indigestion; liquids may offer more relief than tablets.
- Vitamin A, B, D, E, and K supplements help sustain nutritional status and healing.

ACTIVITY

- Physical exercise, as tolerated

NUTRITION

- Low-fat diet

ing, or extensive burns. Sometimes, the cause can't be pinpointed. The patient with acalculous cholecystitis is at greater risk for perforation and gangrene and usually needs immediate surgery.

Chronic cholecystitis also usually results from gallstones. It doesn't cause as much pain as the acute form of the disorder. Other signs and symptoms include heartburn and flatulence, especially after eating fatty foods. Typically, the patient has the disorder for years (usually punctuated with somewhat more acute episodes) and manages it with diet modifications and over-the-counter or prescribed medications. Chronic cholecystitis can result in fibrosis and gallbladder dysfunction.

POTENTIAL COMPLICATIONS
- Infection and sepsis
- Perforation, possibly with peritonitis, abscess, and fistula formation and necrosis

---

TREATMENTS
- Achieving and maintaining appropriate weight

RISK FACTORS
- Obesity
- High-fat, high-calorie diet
- Gender (higher incidence in women)
- Age (adults over age 40)
- Race (higher incidence in whites and Native Americans)
- Multiple pregnancies
- Use of oral contraceptives
- Diabetes mellitus
- Liver and pancreatic disorders

AFTERCARE
- Tell the patient to seek help if the following occur:
  – severe epigastric or chest pain
  – fever
  – nausea and vomiting.

CIRRHOSIS

Cirrhosis is a chronic, progressive disorder in which the liver initially enlarges and then shrinks and hardens, becoming fibrotic and nodular; portal circulatory changes also occur. If diagnosed and treated early, the condition may improve.

Types of cirrhosis include Laënnec's cirrhosis, which stems from alcoholism (the most common cause of cirrhosis in the United States), and postnecrotic cirrhosis, which can result from exposure to toxins. Biliary disease and cardiac disease can also lead to cirrhosis.

In the early stages of cirrhosis, the patient may have no symptoms, although some experience tissue wasting in the upper body, spider angiomas, erythema of the palms, and nausea and vomiting. As the disease progresses, the patient may

TEACHING TOPICS

MEDICATIONS

- Diuretics (such as spirono-lactone) reduce fluid retention in patients with ascites.
- Vitamin A, B, D, E, and K supplements help sustain nutritional status and healing.

ACTIVITY

- Energy-conservation measures and equipment, with possible occupational therapy consult
- Alternating activity with rest to avoid overexertion

NUTRITION

- No alcohol
- Low-salt, low-fat diet
- High-calorie, high-carbohydrate, high-protein diet (possible low-protein diet in advanced stages)
- Restricted fluid intake
- Small, frequent meals (may be better tolerated)
- No raw seafood

develop ascites, bleeding from esophageal varices, spleen enlargement, fetor hepaticus, and encephalitis.

Because of the liver's pivotal role in the breakdown and detoxification of drugs, the patient must not consume any alcohol and must make sure his doctor knows and approves of any drug he takes.

POTENTIAL COMPLICATIONS
- Ascites
- Renal impairment
- Hepatic encephalopathy
- Pulmonary hypertension
- Esophageal varices

TREATMENTS
- Alcohol cessation program for alcoholism
- Vaccinations against hepatitis A and B and influenza virus

RISK FACTORS
- Alcohol abuse
- Drug abuse
- Viral hepatitis
- Right-sided heart failure
- Obstruction or inflammation of the biliary system
- Exposure to certain toxins, pollutants, and chemicals (arsenic, phosphorus, carbon tetrachloride)
- Family history of cirrhosis

AFTERCARE
- Teach the patient and caregiver home total parenteral nutrition administration and safety as needed.
- Tell the patient to:
  – avoid over-the-counter medicines without the doctor's approval, particularly acetaminophen
  – weigh himself daily (at same time, on same scale, with same amount of clothing on), record weights, and report sudden or steady changes.
- Tell the patient to seek help if the following occur:
  – confusion, irritability, or lethargy
  – changes in weight or abdominal girth
  – hallucinations
  – blood in vomitus or stool.

CONSTIPATION

A symptom rather than a disease, constipation can be defined as difficult passage of small, hard stools less than two to three times a week. Deciding whether a patient is constipated, however, rests as much on assessing changes from *his* normal bowel habits—especially if he reports any sudden changes—as it does on any objective criteria.

Several factors influence how quickly food passes through the intestine and how much fluid the bowel absorbs. Poor dietary habits, such as insufficient fiber and water intake; a sedentary lifestyle, which doesn't promote intestinal motility; chronic suppression of the urge to defecate; certain diseases; and the adverse effects of some medications can all interfere with normal bowel function.

TEACHING TOPICS

MEDICATIONS

- Bulk-forming laxatives (such as psyllium, calcium polycarbophil, and methylcellulose) increase the water content and bulk of stool.
- Osmotic laxatives (such as sorbitol and lactulose) increase the water content of stool.
- Surfactant laxatives (such as docusate calcium, potassium, and sodium) soften stools by increasing their fat and water content.
- Stimulant laxatives (such as bisacodyl, cascara, castor oil, phenolphthalein, and senna) promote fluid and electrolyte accumulation in the colon and stimulate intestinal peristalsis.

ACTIVITY

- Regular aerobic exercise (helps stimulate bowel motility)

NUTRITION

- High-fiber diet
- Gradual addition of raw bran as needed
- Adequate hydration
- Warm fluids, including water with lemon juice (may stimulate defecation)

Constipation can result from many disorders and needs careful assessment to determine the underlying cause. It can also cause chronic discomfort, especially for elderly patients. Treatment usually starts with changes in diet, activities, and bowel habits. If the patient needs a laxative, he should first receive a mild, natural (bulk-forming) laxative, progressing if needed to osmotic or surfactant laxatives; he should only receive a stimulant laxative for short-term use during exacerbations.

POTENTIAL COMPLICATIONS
- Hemorrhoids
- Fecal impaction
- Myocardial infarction, cerebrovascular accident, or retinal detachment (from straining)

TREATMENTS
- Tap water or bisacodyl enemas every 3 to 4 days
- Suppositories as ordered
- Manual removal of impaction
- Bowel training
- Biofeedback for appropriate muscle and sphincter contraction

RISK FACTORS
- Low-fiber diet
- Inadequate fluid intake
- Sedentary lifestyle
- Regular suppression of the urge to defecate
- Diseases and conditions (some congenital diseases, GI disorders and lesions, neurologic disorders, liver disorders, endocrine disorders, pelvic floor dyssynergia, mesenteric artery ischemia)
- Drugs (analgesics, antacids, anticholinergics, anticonvulsants, antidepressants, antipsychotics, antihypertensives, antiparkinsonian medications, calcium channel blockers, diuretics, opiates)

AFTERCARE
- If the patient has limited mobility (after surgery or from disability or debilitation), provide a bedside commode to encourage quick response to the urge to defecate.
- Tell the patient to seek help if the following occur:
  – abdominal pain and severe cramping
  – continued constipation after treatment
  – diarrhea.

DIVERTICULAR DISEASE

In diverticular disease, small, bulging mucosal pouches (diverticula) form on the walls of the GI tract. They can form almost anywhere along the tract, from the esophagus to the colon, but usually occur in the sigmoid colon. They seem to form at weak areas along the intestinal wall, perhaps from pressure within the intestine. If a diverticulum contains all layers of the intestinal wall—mucosa, submucosa, and muscle—it's called a true diverticulum; a false diverticulum doesn't contain the muscle layer.

Two forms of diverticular disease exist. A patient with diverticulosis has diverticula (typically found during various diagnostic tests or surgery for another condition) but no other signs. A patient with diverticulitis has one or more inflamed diverticula. The inflammation usually results from microperforation of a diverticulum that's blocked with trapped thickened fecal material. Diverticulitis typically

TEACHING TOPICS

MEDICATIONS

- Antibiotics (such as gentamicin, clindamycin, aztreonam, cefoxitin, ticarcillin, and ciprofloxacin) combat infection.
- Antibacterials (such as metronidazole) combat anaerobic bacterial infection.
- Bulk-forming laxatives (such as methylcellulose and psyllium) increase the water content and bulk of stool.

ACTIVITY

- No isometric activities (straining, coughing, lifting) to avoid increasing intra-abdominal pressure and aggravating symptoms

NUTRITION

- High-fiber diet
- No nuts, seeds, corn, or similar hard foods (controversial)
- Psyllium or cellulose products (to increase fiber content)
- Adequate hydration

has a sudden onset, with abdominal pain in the left lower quadrant, fever, and possibly nausea and vomiting. If the swollen diverticulum aggravates the bladder, the patient may experience urinary frequency and pain on urination.

Treatment takes place either in the hospital or home with I.V. or oral antibiotics or antibacterial agents or a combination of the two. If the inflammation doesn't resolve or perforation or obstruction occurs, the patient may need surgery.

POTENTIAL COMPLICATIONS
- Inflammation
- Infection
- Perforation
- Bleeding
- Obstruction of the bowel

TREATMENTS
- Achieving and maintaining appropriate weight
- Smoking cessation (smoke irritates gastric mucosa)
- Colon resection if perforation or obstruction occurs or inflammation doesn't resolve

RISK FACTORS
- Culture (higher incidence in developed countries, including United Kingdom, France, United States, and Australia)
- Age (adults over age 50)
- Chronic constipation
- Obesity

AFTERCARE
- Teach the patient techniques for managing pain.
- Tell the patient to seek help if the following occur:
  – unusual diarrhea or constipation
  – mucus or blood in stool
  – fever
  – abdominal pain or distention
  – urinary frequency or cloudy, foul-smelling urine.

GASTROESOPHAGEAL REFLUX DISEASE

Gastroesophageal reflux disease (GERD) is the backflow of gastric contents past the lower esophageal sphincter (LES) into the distal end of the esophagus. Mild forms of the disorder produce occasional attacks that can be controlled with over-the-counter antacids. More severe disease can lead to precancerous changes in the epithelium of the esophagus from repeated exposure to the irritating contents of the lower digestive tract and may require surgery. Although incidence of GERD continues to rise, newer over-the-counter medications allow patients with milder forms of the disease to control their own symptoms without further treatment.

Normally, the LES prevents backflow of gastric contents; GERD results when the LES fails to perform this function, either because of incompetence or another cause. Predisposing factors include obesity, pregnancy, tobacco use, surgery, or intubation of the esophagus and stomach.

Symptoms can come on gradually or suddenly. Heartburn, the classic symptom, results from acid in the esophagus. Other indications include difficult and

TEACHING TOPICS

MEDICATIONS

- Antacids (such as magnesium-aluminum hydroxide, aluminum hydroxide, and calcium carbonate) inhibit acid secretion.
- Proton pump inhibitors (such as omeprazole) inhibit gastric acid secretion.
- GI stimulants (such as cisapride) promote rapid emptying of stomach contents.
- Histamine$_2$-receptor antagonists (such as cimetidine, nizatidine, and ranitidine) decrease gastric acid secretion.

ACTIVITY

- As tolerated
- No isometric activities (straining, coughing, lifting) to avoid increasing intra-abdominal pressure and aggravating symptoms

NUTRITION

- No fatty foods, chocolate, peppermint, onions, or other foods known to bring on symptoms
- Small, bland, nutritious meals
- Eating slowly and chewing food thoroughly (to help prevent bloating)
- Staying upright for 2 to 3 hours after eating
- Chewing gum and sucking hard candy (increases salivation, which may soothe esophageal irritation)
- Adequate hydration

painful swallowing, excessive salivation, an acid or salty taste in the mouth (water brash), a bloated feeling after eating even a small amount of food, and the sensation of food remaining stuck in the esophagus after swallowing.

Drug treatment with antacids and histamine$_2$-receptor antagonists aims to control symptoms by neutralizing gastric contents. Despite such treatment, some patients continue to have symptoms of GERD; others may gain symptomatic relief but continue to have negative epithelial changes, which can result in Barrett's epithelium. Such responses indicate that other factors besides acid may contribute to GERD.

POTENTIAL COMPLICATIONS
- Stricture
- Ulceration
- Short esophagus
- Barrett's epithelium
- Aspiration pneumonia

TREATMENTS
- Achieving and maintaining appropriate weight
- Smoking cessation
- Elevating the head of the bed about 6" (15 cm) with wooden blocks or a wedge under the mattress

RISK FACTORS
- Obesity
- Tobacco use
- Pregnancy
- Hiatal hernia
- Esophageal or gastric surgery
- Prolonged vomiting
- Prolonged GI intubation

AFTERCARE
- Offer the patient emotional support and (if needed) suggest counseling.
- Tell the patient to seek help if the following occur:
  – fever
  – wheezing
  – coughing
  – painful or difficult swallowing.

HEMORRHOIDS

A common complaint, hemorrhoids are believed to be veins in the anal area that swell and engorge from chronic straining to defecate. Prolonged sitting, standing, and lifting can aggravate symptoms from existing hemorrhoids, but they aren't believed to contribute to their development.

Hemorrhoids are classified as first through fourth degree. First- and second-degree internal hemorrhoids bulge into the rectum and are covered by rectal mucosa; second-degree hemorrhoids may prolapse painlessly and spontaneously return to the anal canal after defecation. Straining and passing hard stools can push hemorrhoids through the anus, creating third- or fourth-degree external hemorrhoids—a vascular mass that can interfere with normal defecation and cause bleeding, thromboses, infection, and pain. Third-degree hemorrhoids must be manually reduced, and fourth-degree hemorrhoids can't be reduced and remain prolapsed at all times.

TEACHING TOPICS

MEDICATIONS

- Bulk-forming laxatives (such as psyllium, calcium polycarbophil, and methylcellulose) increase the water content and bulk of stool.
- Surfactant laxatives (such as docusate calcium, potassium, and sodium) soften stool by increasing fat and water content.
- Topical steroids (such as hydrocortisone) help reduce inflammation and swelling.
- Topical anesthetics (such as dibucaine and tetracaine) relieve pain and itching.

ACTIVITY

- Regular aerobic exercise (to stimulate bowel motility)
- No sitting or standing for long periods
- No sitting on the toilet for prolonged periods or straining during defecation

NUTRITION

- High-fiber diet
- Adequate hydration

Many patients assume that any painful or bleeding anal lesions are hemorrhoids and require careful assessment to determine whether they have hemorrhoids or another disorder, such as anal fissures or anorectal abscesses or fistulas. Physical examination and questioning about pain, bleeding, protrusion, itching, and normal bowel habits can lead to a differential diagnosis.

Treatment for small, uncomplicated hemorrhoids includes a high-fiber diet, adequate hydration, regular exercise, bulk-forming and surfactant laxatives, and topical steroid cream. Proper hygiene can improve anal itching.

POTENTIAL COMPLICATIONS
- Hemorrhage
- Infection

TREATMENTS
- Warm (not hot) sitz baths
- Thorough cleaning of perianal area after defecation (with gentle wipes, not harsh toilet paper)
- Warm or cold packs to the anal area (both relieve pain; cold packs help reduce hemorrhoids)
- Sclerotherapy
- Rubber band ligation
- Cryosurgery
- Laser surgery
- Hemorrhoidectomy

RISK FACTORS
- Family history of hemorrhoids
- Pregnancy
- Straining during defecation
- Heart failure
- Cirrhosis with portal hypertension

AFTERCARE
- Tell the patient to sit on cushions or pillows—not a rubber doughnut—to help ease pain in the anal area.
- Tell the patient to seek help if the following occur:
  – constipation
  – urge to defecate, but inability to do so.

HEPATITIS, VIRAL

An inflammation of the liver, viral hepatitis in the United States typically results from infection with hepatitis A, B, or C. Infection with hepatitis D (delta hepatitis) and E as well as with hepatitis F- and G-related agents occurs more commonly in countries other than the United States.

Although the means of transmission vary, all types of viral hepatitis are infectious. Infection with hepatitis A usually occurs through the fecal-oral route. Infection with hepatitis B and C typically occurs from direct exchange of contaminated blood (for instance, from shared needles or blood transfusions), although infection with hepatitis B can also occur from contact with human secretions and feces. Hepatitis D occurs only in conjunction with hepatitis B.

In almost all cases of hepatitis, the patient has a low-grade fever, feels nauseous, and generally doesn't feel well. His liver becomes swollen and tender, and

TEACHING TOPICS

MEDICATIONS

- Vitamin K supplements help prevent bleeding.
- Immune serums (such as immune globulin) provide passive immunity by increasing the antibody titer.
- Hepatitis A or B vaccine provides active immunization.
- Antiviral, immunoregulators (such as interferon) stop viral growth (used in hepatitis B and C infections).
- Histamine$_2$-receptor antagonists (such as cimetidine, nizatidine, ranitidine, and famotidine) decrease gastric acid secretion.

ACTIVITY

- Possibly extremely restricted (possibly bed rest), with progression as tolerated
- Regular aerobic exercise as tolerated; no overexertion

NUTRITION

- Low-fat, high-carbohydrate diet
- Small, frequent meals (may be better tolerated)
- Adequate hydration
- No alcoholic beverages for up to a year after attack

jaundice develops. The patient with hepatitis A usually has an uncomplicated recovery. Hepatitis B may take up to 6 months to develop and can result in chronic hepatitis, acute liver failure, or cirrhosis; years later, the patient may develop hepatocellular carcinoma. Although hepatitis C infection usually isn't as acute as infection from hepatitis A or B, it can result in chronic infection. Hepatitis D (in conjunction with hepatitis B) can result in acute hepatitis or cirrhosis of the liver.

POTENTIAL COMPLICATIONS
- Fulminant hepatitis, liver failure
- Chronic hepatitis (hepatitis B and C)
- Cirrhosis, hepatocellular carcinoma (years later) (hepatitis B)
- Liver fibrosis (hepatitis C)

TREATMENTS
- Smoking cessation
- Liver transplantation in end-stage liver disease

RISK FACTORS
- Hepatitis A: ingestion of contaminated milk, food, or water; poor sanitation
- Hepatitis B: high-risk behaviors (unprotected sex, needle sharing, tattooing), being born to an infected mother, transfusion of contaminated blood and blood products
- Hepatitis C: high-risk behaviors (needle sharing, tattooing, unprotected sex [risk lower than with hepatitis B]), transfusion of contaminated blood and blood products

AFTERCARE
- Tell the patient to:
  – weigh himself daily
  – inform all health care personnel
  – inform potential sex partners and practice safer sex.
- Tell the patient to seek help if the following occur:
  – persistent vomiting and deepening jaundice
  – changes in level of consciousness
  – confusion
  – personality changes
  – flapping of the hands (asterixis)
  – blood in vomitus, stool, or urine
  – unusual bruising and prolonged bleeding
  – abdominal edema
  – weight gain.

HIATAL HERNIA

A hernia is the protrusion of all or part of an organ through the wall of the cavity that normally contains it. In hiatal hernia, a weakness in the diaphragmatic opening allows the lower esophageal sphincter (LES) and part of the stomach to protrude into the chest. In sliding hiatal hernia, the LES, the junction of the esophagus and stomach, and the upper stomach slip up into the thorax. In a rolling hiatal hernia, the LES and junction remain below the diaphragm, but part or all of the stomach slips up into the chest.

Most hiatal hernias are sliding hernias, which can cause esophageal reflux and related chest pain. A rolling hiatal hernia usually doesn't cause esophageal reflux.

TEACHING TOPICS

MEDICATIONS

- Antacids (such as magnesium-aluminum hydroxide, aluminum hydroxides, and calcium carbonates) inhibit acid secretion.
- Proton pump inhibitors (such as omeprazole) inhibit gastric acid secretion.
- GI stimulants (such as cisapride) promote rapid emptying of stomach contents.
- Histamine$_2$-receptor antagonists (such as cimetidine, nizatidine, and ranitidine) decrease gastric acid secretion.

ACTIVITY

- Regular, gentle exercise
- No isometric activities (straining, coughing, lifting) to avoid increasing intra-abdominal pressure and aggravating symptoms

NUTRITION

- No foods known to bring on symptoms
- Small, bland, nutritious meals
- Eating slowly and chewing food thoroughly (to help prevent bloating)
- Staying upright for 2 to 3 hours after eating

The patient may instead feel very full even after eating small amounts and have difficulty breathing or chest pain that grows worse when he lies down.

Some patients have few if any symptoms and may need no more treatment than careful attention to the timing and contents of their meals and perhaps antacids. Others may need more comprehensive medications, perhaps surgery.

POTENTIAL COMPLICATIONS
- Gastroesophageal reflux disease
- Aspiration pneumonia
- Obstruction
- Strangulation
- Volvulus

TREATMENTS
- Achieving and maintaining appropriate weight
- Smoking cessation
- Elevating the head of the bed about 6" (15 cm) with wooden blocks or a wedge under the mattress

RISK FACTORS
- Age (adults age 50 and older)
- Gender (higher incidence in women)
- Obesity
- Pregnancy
- Congenital weakness of the diaphragmatic opening around the esophagus
- Abdominal or chest injury

AFTERCARE
- Tell the patient to avoid restrictive clothing such as girdles.
- Tell the patient to seek help if the following occur:
  – increased difficulty swallowing
  – nausea and vomiting
  – fever
  – difficulty breathing.

INFLAMMATORY BOWEL DISEASE

The two most common inflammatory bowel diseases are ulcerative colitis and Crohn's disease. Although the exact cause of inflammatory bowel disease isn't known, genetics seems to play a role. Some patients have signs and symptoms of both diseases.

In ulcerative colitis, inflammation affects the mucosa and submucosa of the intestinal tract. The ulcerated bowel wall appears swollen and congested, with tiny tears that ooze blood and may develop into abscesses. This blood causes rectal bleeding, one of the hallmark signs of ulcerative colitis. Other signs and symptoms include abdominal cramping, tenesmus (painful spasms of the anal sphincter), and rectal urgency; early morning rectal urgency and bloody nocturnal bowel movements also differentiate ulcerative colitis from Crohn's disease. Later stages of ulcerative colitis can cause fever, weight loss, and anemia.

TEACHING TOPICS

MEDICATIONS

- Antispasmodics reduce cramping in mild disease.
- Antidiarrheals inhibit diarrhea.
- Aminosalicylates decrease inflammation and swelling.
- Steroids decrease inflammation and swelling.
- Immunosuppressants can be used to decrease inflammation when steroids don't.
- Antibacterials prevent or combat infection in Crohn's disease.
- Antilipemics help control watery diarrhea from malabsorption of bile acid in Crohn's disease patients who've had an ileal resection.

ACTIVITY

- As tolerated, with extra rest as needed
- Bed rest during exacerbations as needed

NUTRITION

- Fiber content based on patient's tolerance and severity of disease
- High-calorie, high-protein diet, with nutritional consult
- No foods that aggravate symptoms
- Small, frequent meals (may help prevent immediate, distressing urge to defecate)
- Adequate fluids
- Low-oxalate diet (for Crohn's disease patients who develop steatorrhea and hyperoxaluria)

Crohn's disease causes patchy, not continuous, bowel inflammation that affects all layers of the bowel wall; granulomas and fissures may also develop. The disease can affect the entire GI tract but mostly involves the terminal ileum. Other signs and symptoms typically include perianal lesions and inflammatory conditions of the skin, eyes, joints, and liver and may include arthritis.

POTENTIAL COMPLICATIONS
- Fulminant colitis (in ulcerative colitis)
- Toxic megacolon with perforation and peritonitis (in ulcerative colitis)
- Intestinal obstruction and perforation (in Crohn's disease)
- Perianal abscesses, fistulas, and fissures (in Crohn's disease)
- Electrolyte imbalance (in both)
- Dehydration, malnutrition, and anemia (in both)

TREATMENTS
- Perianal area care daily and after each bowel movement (washing with moisturized soap and warm water and applying ointment or gel to prevent excoriation)
- Stress management and relaxation techniques and biofeedback
- Surgery, if necessary, to treat complications

RISK FACTORS
- Family history of ulcerative colitis or Crohn's disease
- Age (young adults and occasionally teenagers)
- Race (higher incidence in whites, particularly Jews)

AFTERCARE
- Teach the patient to use and care for ostomy, appliances, and equipment.
- Tell the patient to:
  – weigh himself daily
  – keep a record of bowel movements
  – recognize that stress can cause exacerbations
  – avoid over-the-counter drugs without the doctor's permission.
- Tell the patient to seek help if the following occur:
  – abdominal pain unrelieved by approved analgesics
  – unusual bloating and distention
  – vomiting
  – increased diarrhea
  – bloody stool
  – hard, tight abdomen.

PANCREATITIS, CHRONIC

Unlike acute pancreatitis, which is generally reversible, chronic pancreatitis is a progressive, irreversible inflammatory disease. As it progresses, the pancreas becomes damaged, fibrotic, and dysfunctional. It may develop after an initial acute episode or after recurrent acute attacks.

The most common cause of chronic pancreatitis in most Western cultures is excessive alcohol intake. Other causes include cystic fibrosis, some autoimmune disorders, and hyperparathyroidism. The most common symptom is alternately severe or dull, recurrent or continuous abdominal pain that can radiate to the back and that worsens after eating. Many patients lose weight as the disease progresses, partly because eating exacerbates the pain and partly because inflammation of the pancreas leads to reduced output of pancreatic enzymes, resulting in malabsorption of food and malnutrition. If the pancreas also loses the ability to

TEACHING TOPICS

MEDICATIONS

- Digestive enzymes (such as pancreatin and pancrelipase) help digest proteins, carbohydrates, and fat.
- Histamine$_2$-receptor antagonists (such as cimetidine, nizatidine, ranitidine, and famotidine) decrease gastric acid secretion and raise gastric and duodenal pH.
- Oral antidiabetic drugs (such as chlorpropamide and tolbutamide) promote the release of insulin from pancreatic cells.
- Antidiabetic drugs (such as insulin) promote glucose entry into cells.
- Narcotic or nonnarcotic analgesics help relieve pain.

ACTIVITY

- Progressive walking program, alternating activity with rest (patient may be malnourished and in pain)
- Energy-conservation measures and equipment, with possible occupational therapy consult

NUTRITION

- Healthy diet based on recommended portions from the food pyramid
- Low-fat, low-fiber diet as needed
- Vitamin B$_{12}$ supplements as needed
- Small, frequent meals (may be easier to digest)
- Diabetic diet as needed (possible nutritional consult)
- Resting after meals (to aid digestion)
- Possible antioxidants and zinc supplements (controversial)
- No alcohol

produce insulin, the patient may develop diabetes mellitus. Chronic pancreatitis also causes steatorrhea (stools with a high fat content).

Medical management includes controlling pain, eliminating the cause of the condition, and replacing the digestive enzymes and insulin the pancreas can no longer adequately provide. If the disorder resulted from excessive alcohol, management includes stopping alcohol intake, which may also stop the patient's pain. If pain can't be controlled or if complications arise, the patient may need surgery. The specific surgical procedure depends on the underlying cause.

POTENTIAL COMPLICATIONS
- Pancreatic pseudocyst
- GI or biliary tract obstruction
- Infection
- Fistula formation

TREATMENTS
- Alcohol cessation program for alcoholism

RISK FACTORS
- Gender (higher incidence in men)
- Excessive alcohol consumption (more than ½ cup a day for more than 6 years in association with a high-fat diet)
- Obstruction of pancreatic drainage by trauma or tumors
- Cystic fibrosis
- Some autoimmune disorders
- Hyperparathyroidism

AFTERCARE
- If the patient becomes addicted to narcotic analgesics, he may need treatment for narcotic addiction.
- Tell the patient to avoid crowds and people with infections.
- Tell the patient to seek help if the following occur:
  – sudden, severe abdominal pain
  – nausea and vomiting persist
  – fever
  – blood glucose level hard to control.

PEPTIC ULCER DISEASE

A break or erosion in the mucous membrane, peptic ulcers occur in the lining of the stomach (gastric) or duodenum (duodenal). Of the two types, gastric ulcers are generally harder to treat, have a much higher incidence of malignancy, and can result from either *Helicobacter pylori* infection (more than half) or non-steroidal anti-inflammatory drug (NSAID) use. In contrast, duodenal ulcers rarely become malignant and almost always result from *H. pylori* infection. Predisposing factors include cigarette smoking and possibly diet and stress, although the role of stress and diet is controversial.

Gastric ulcers typically cause burning or gnawing epigastric pain in the left upper quadrant that worsens on eating. Other signs include nausea and vomiting, either occult or frank bleeding in vomitus, and occult blood in stools. Duodenal ulcers cause burning, gnawing epigastric pain relieved by eating or taking antacids.

TEACHING TOPICS

MEDICATIONS

- Antacids (such as magnesium-aluminum hydroxides, aluminum hydroxides, and calcium carbonates) inhibit gastric acid secretion and provide relief from indigestion; liquids may offer more relief than tablets.
- Proton pump inhibitors (such as omeprazole and lansoprazole) inhibit gastric acid secretion.
- Histamine$_2$-receptor antagonists (such as cimetidine, nizatidine, and ranitidine) decrease gastric acid secretion.
- Antibiotics (such as tetracycline and clarithromycin) combat infection.
- Antibacterials (such as metronidazole) combat infection.

ACTIVITY

- As tolerated

NUTRITION

- No foods known to bring on symptoms
- Small, frequent meals (may help minimize symptoms)
- No alcohol

Depending on the cause, the patient's response to treatment, and the extent of damage, treatment can range from antacid and antibiotic therapy to sometimes-extensive surgery. Despite treatment, many peptic ulcers tend to recur.

A third type of peptic ulcer, a stress ulcer can develop in a patient who has experienced extensive trauma (particularly head trauma), received severe burns, or been critically ill. These acute gastric erosions don't cause symptoms until they hemorrhage.

POTENTIAL COMPLICATIONS
- Hemorrhage and shock
- Perforation and peritonitis
- Pyloric stenosis

TREATMENTS
- Smoking cessation and avoiding second-hand smoke
- Surgery, if necessary, to treat severe bleeding, obstruction, or perforation

RISK FACTORS
- Family history of gastric or duodenal ulcers
- Gender (higher incidence in men)
- Stress (controversial)
- Infection
- Some medications (salicylates, NSAIDs, steroids)

AFTERCARE
- Tell the patient to:
  – take the entire course of medication, even if symptoms improve, or the ulcer may not completely heal
  – practice stress management techniques as appropriate.
- Tell the patient to seek help if the following occur:
  – sudden onset of excruciating epigastric pain
  – bright red or coffee-ground vomitus
  – blood in stools
  – fever.

ADRENAL INSUFFICIENCY

Adrenal insufficiency occurs when the adrenal glands fail to produce enough cortisol and aldosterone. Atrophy or destruction of the adrenal tissue itself results in Addison's disease (primary adrenal insufficiency). A lack of corticotropin, which is produced in the pituitary and affected by the hypothalamus, results in secondary adrenal insufficiency.

In Addison's disease, adrenal tissue destruction most commonly results from an immune response. Infections such as tuberculosis, histoplasmosis, coccidioidomycosis, and cytomegalovirus can also cause adrenal damage. Drugs such as mitotane, ketoconazole, rifampin, phenytoin, and phenobarbital can also destroy adrenal tissue.

In most cases of Addison's disease, the patient slowly develops such signs and symptoms as weight loss, excessive tiredness, nausea and vomiting, decrease in

TEACHING TOPICS

MEDICATIONS

- Steroids (such as cortisone, hydrocortisone, prednisone, and fludrocortisone) replace the glucocorticoids the body can't make.

ACTIVITY

- Regular aerobic activity (helps prevent muscle wasting and improve bone strength)
- Low-impact activities (walking, swimming) to decrease risk of bone fracture
- Alternating activity with rest to prevent overexertion
- No exercise in extremely hot, humid weather (to avoid overworking the adrenal glands)

NUTRITION

- High-calorie, high-carbohydrate, high-protein diet
- Vitamin supplements

body hair, hyperpigmentation, and postural hypotension. Treatment consists of replacing adrenal hormones. However, acute stresses—such as pregnancy, trauma, infection, and emotional upset—can trigger a critical adrenal hormone deficiency, leading to addisonian crisis. Without prompt treatment, addisonian crisis can lead to coma and death.

The most common causes of secondary adrenal insufficiency include bilateral adrenalectomy, hemorrhagic infarction and necrosis of the adrenal glands, hypopituitarism, and corticotropin suppression. Typically, the patient with secondary insufficiency produces enough aldosterone but not enough cortisol. Treatment consists of cortisol replacement.

POTENTIAL COMPLICATIONS
- Addisonian crisis (in Addison's disease)
- Osteoporosis

TREATMENTS
- Stress management and relaxation techniques

RISK FACTORS
- Sudden cessation of established steroid therapy
- Tuberculosis
- Acquired immunodeficiency disease
- Other endocrine disorders
- Adrenalectomy
- Certain medications (mitotane, ketoconazole, rifampin, phenytoin, and phenobarbital)

AFTERCARE
- Tell the patient to:
  – wear medical identification
  – always keep an emergency hydrocortisone kit on hand and know how to use it
  – inform all doctors, dentists, and other health care professionals of his condition.
- Tell the female patient that pregnancy will be high risk.
- Tell the patient to seek help if the following occur:
  – fever
  – respiratory infection
  – delayed wound healing.
- Reinforce the doctor's instructions on increasing oral steroid dosage when the patient is sick.

CUSHING'S SYNDROME

Also called hypercortisolism, Cushing's syndrome is the cluster of effects that occur when the adrenal glands produce excessive levels of adrenocortical hormones. The syndrome can result from a benign or malignant cortisol-secreting adrenal tumor. More commonly, the syndrome occurs when the pituitary produces too much corticotropin, which in turn stimulates the adrenal glands to release cortisol (Cushing's disease). However, most cases of Cushing's syndrome result from long-term steroid replacement therapy or excessive steroid administration.

Cushing's syndrome causes distinctive signs, including the characteristic rounded moon face, thinning hair on top of the head, and acne and male-pattern hair growth on the rest of the face. Other signs include a "buffalo hump" behind the neck, an obese abdomen, thin extremities (from muscle wasting and weak-

TEACHING TOPICS

MEDICATIONS

- Adrenal blocking agents (such as metyrapone, aminoglutethimide, ketoconazole, and mitotane) decrease cortisol levels.
- Agents that reduce corticotropin production (such as cyproheptadine, somatostatin, and bromocriptine) indirectly decrease cortisol levels.
- Steroids (such as prednisone) following surgical removal of the adrenals replace natural steroids the body can no longer produce.
- Diuretics (such as spironolactone) help regulate potassium and sodium and block androgen receptor sites, decreasing hirsutism, oiliness, and acne.

ACTIVITY

- Regular aerobic activity (helps prevent muscle wasting and improve bone strength)
- Low-impact activities (walking, swimming) to decrease risk of bone fracture
- Alternating activity with rest to prevent overexertion

NUTRITION

- High-potassium diet
- Low-sodium, low-carbohydrate, low-calorie diet

ness), and ankle and foot swelling. The skin becomes thin and bruises easily, and striae develop on the trunk and legs. The patient has slowed healing, poor resistance to infection, hyperglycemia, and osteoporosis. The patient may also become emotionally labile, grow confused, have diminished mental ability, or develop depression or bipolar disorder.

POTENTIAL COMPLICATIONS
- Hypokalemia
- Heart failure
- Arrhythmias
- Infections and sepsis
- Peptic ulcer
- Osteoporosis and fractures
- Diabetes mellitus

TREATMENTS
- Surgery, radiation treatment, or drug therapy (to restore hormone balance)
- Achieving and maintaining appropriate weight
- Possible emergency hydrocortisone injection (if treatment results in dangerously low cortisol levels)
- Stress reduction and relaxation techniques

RISK FACTORS
- Gender (higher incidence in women)
- Chronic or excessive use of steroids (cortisone, prednisone)

AFTERCARE
- Tell the patient to:
  – carry and know how to use an emergency hydrocortisone kit (as needed)
  – weigh himself daily, record weights, and report sudden or steady changes
  – keep his home well lighted, use handrails, remove throw rugs, and take measures to help prevent falls
  – wear medical identification
  – avoid stopping or changing medications without the doctor's approval
  – expect emotional lability.
- Tell the patient to seek help if the following occur:
  – sudden or steady weight gain or loss
  – difficulty breathing
  – pain or swelling after a fall
  – fever.

DIABETES MELLITUS

Diabetes mellitus (DM) occurs when either the pancreas doesn't produce enough insulin or the cells aren't able to use available insulin, resulting in abnormal metabolism of carbohydrates, fats, and proteins. About 10.3 million people in the United States have been diagnosed with the disease, and estimates suggest that roughly the same number have undiagnosed DM. The disease can occur as type 1 DM or type 2 DM. Diabetes can also be categorized as secondary (resulting from other diseases or medications), impaired glucose tolerance, or gestational (which typically resolves after delivery).

The hyperglycemia that results from DM can cause damage throughout the body, affecting the heart and blood vessels, brain and nerves, eyes, kidneys, digestion, and immune and healing responses. Specifically, DM underlies many new cases of coronary artery disease, blindness, renal failure, and lower-extremity amputations. Death can also result from such blood glucose crises as diabetic ke-

TEACHING TOPICS

MEDICATIONS

- Insulins (such as insulin lispro, regular, NPH, lente, and ultralente) lower blood glucose levels by promoting the transport of glucose into cells, preventing cells from using proteins and fats for energy.
- Oral antidiabetic drugs (such as tolbutamide, chlorpropamide, glipizide, glyburide, metformin, acarbose, and troglitazone) stimulate insulin production in the pancreas and increase the number of insulin receptor sites.

ACTIVITY

- Regular aerobic exercise (to strengthen muscle, bone, and cardiovascular system)

NUTRITION

- Readily available sugar sources (such as hard candy)
- Diabetes exchange diet, adjusted as needed to meet age requirements and increased activity needs (nutritional consult)

toacidosis (DKA), hypoglycemia (from an insulin overdose or from not eating after taking insulin), and hyperosmolar nonketotic coma.

National efforts to encourage healthier diets and promote weight loss and exercise can help decrease the overall incidence of type 2 DM.

POTENTIAL COMPLICATIONS
- DKA (usually in type 1 DM)
- Hyperosmolar nonketotic coma (type 2 DM)
- Hypoglycemia
- Retinopathy
- Neuropathy
- Cardiovascular disease
- Kidney disease
- Infections

TREATMENTS
- Insulin administration
- Blood glucose monitoring
- Achieving and maintaining appropriate weight
- Glucagon administration (to treat hypoglycemia)
- Foot and skin care
- Toenail, corn, and callus care as needed (by a diabetes nurse or podiatrist)

RISK FACTORS
- Family history of diabetes mellitus
- Obesity
- High-fat, high-calorie diet
- Decreased physical activity
- Stress

AFTERCARE
- Teach the patient how to:
  – administer insulin
  – monitor blood glucose level.
- Teach patient or caregiver to:
  – administer glucagon
  – test urine for ketones
  – adjust insulin dosage, activities, and fluids on sick days.
- Tell the patient to:
  – wear medical identification
  – receive regular eye examinations by an ophthalmologist.
- Tell patient to seek help if the following occur:
  – a blood glucose level above 200 mg/dl
  – fever and chills
  – excessive thirst or urination
  – lethargy
  – shakiness
  – nausea.

GOUT

Gout is a metabolic bone disorder in which uric acid crystals accumulate in the tissues and joints, particularly the first metatarsal joint of the big toe, causing pain. In some patients the crystals form tophi—sharp, pointed clusters that irritate the synovium and cause inflammation and tremendous pain.

Primary gout is caused by a hereditary defect in purine metabolism that results in high levels of uric acid in the blood. However, not all patients with high levels of uric acid develop gout. What's more, some patients with normal uric acid levels suffer from attacks of gout.

Secondary gout causes the same signs and symptoms as primary gout but can result from blood and renal disorders, certain medications (such as aspirin, thiazide diuretics, and antineoplastics), lead poisoning, alcohol intoxication, and starvation.

The patient usually has his first attack of gout in his 40s. The affected joint suddenly becomes red, swollen, and painful, and the patient may develop a fever

TEACHING TOPICS

MEDICATIONS

- NSAIDs (such as indomethacin) decrease inflammation and pain.
- Steroids (such as prednisone) decrease inflammation.
- Antigout agents (such as colchicine and allopurinol) decrease uric acid crystal deposits or uric acid production, reducing inflammation and pain.
- Uricosurics (such as probenecid) increase uric acid excretion.

ACTIVITY

- Possible bed rest during severe attacks, with the affected joint elevated
- Use of crutches or a walker as needed, with physical therapy consult for safe use
- Range-of-motion exercises when inflammation decreases

NUTRITION

- Adequate fluid intake (to flush uric acid through the kidneys and discourage calculi formation)
- No alcohol (may bring on an attack)
- Possible low-purine diet (controversial)

and tachycardia. The attack typically subsides after a week, leaving the skin itching and peeling. The patient may not have another attack for years or may experience four or more attacks annually. Eventually, the patient will have restricted movement in the affected joints and may develop tophi on the ears, knuckles, wrists, elbows, knees, and feet. He may also develop hypertension and atherosclerosis.

To help prevent attacks, the patient may receive prophylactic treatment with antigout medications or uricosurics, or he may instead receive nonsteroidal anti-inflammatory drugs (NSAIDs) or antigout medications at the first sign of pain. Some patients may need joints replaced.

POTENTIAL COMPLICATIONS
- Gouty arthritis
- Renal calculi
- Infection
- Hypertension

TREATMENTS
- Achieving and maintaining appropriate weight
- Ice packs (to reduce inflammation during an attack)

RISK FACTORS
- Gender (much higher incidence in men)
- Family history of gout
- Chemotherapy
- Radiation therapy
- Some blood and renal diseases

AFTERCARE
- Tell the patient to avoid aspirin, thiazide diuretics, and nicotinic acid (these increase uric acid in the blood).
- Tell the patient to seek help if the following occur:
  - flank pain
  - inability to void
  - fever and chills
  - pain in affected joint not relieved by usual measures.

HYPERLIPIDEMIA

Lipids are naturally occurring fats that the body uses to produce hormones, repair cells, and make vitamin D. However, high levels of the lipids cholesterol and triglycerides contribute to an estimated half of the 600,000 deaths that result annually in the United States from coronary artery disease (CAD).

Lipids are carried throughout the body in lipoproteins. Two types of lipoproteins, low-density lipoprotein (LDL) and high-density lipoprotein (HDL), play a major role in CAD. Normally, LDL helps transport cholesterol to body cells. However, in the presence of free radicals, oxidized LDL contributes to plaque formation and buildup in arterial walls; triglycerides also play a role in plaque formation. Blood flow through these narrowed, atherosclerotic arteries slows, contributing to CAD. Blood flow eventually stops when plaque buildup blocks the artery completely or when clots of calcified material break off from the arterial wall and block an artery, potentially resulting in myocardial infarction (MI). In

TEACHING TOPICS

MEDICATIONS

- LDL-lowering antilipemics (such as cholestyramine, colestipol, atorvastatin, fluvastatin, lovastatin, pravastatin, and simvastatin) either promote excretion of cholesterol in stool or reduce cholesterol production, lowering serum LDL.
- Estrogens (such as conjugated estrogen, estropipate, ethinyl estradiol, medroxyprogesterone acetate, and transdermal estradiol) help maintain bone mass and lower cholesterol in postmenopausal women.
- HDL-raising antilipemics (such as nicotinic acid and gemfibrozil) increase HDL and decrease triglycerides.

ACTIVITY

- 20 to 30 minutes of regular aerobic exercise each day (to achieve and maintain appropriate weight, lower heart rate and blood pressure, and increase HDL levels)

NUTRITION

- American Heart Association diet for patients with high cholesterol levels (no more than 20% of total calories from fat [no more than 7% from saturated fat]); more than 55% of calories from carbohydrates (40% to 45% for older women), especially grains, vegetables, and fruits
- Diet that contains about 15% protein
- No more than 200 mg/day of cholesterol
- High-fiber diet

contrast to LDL, HDL helps remove cholesterol from artery walls and take it back to the liver, helping combat atherosclerosis.

One of the main causes of hyperlipidemia is the high-calorie, high-fat, high-protein, low-fiber diet typical in the United States. More than 50% of adults in the United States have cholesterol levels over 200 mg/dl, compared with less than 10% in countries where people typically eat a low-fat, low-protein, high-fiber diet.

Treatment, then, focuses on lowering LDL, triglyceride, and cholesterol levels and raising HDL levels through diet, increased activity, avoidance of tobacco, and moderate alcohol use. Drug treatment includes antilipemics.

POTENTIAL COMPLICATIONS
- CAD
- Stroke
- MI

TREATMENTS
- Achieving and maintaining appropriate weight
- Smoking cessation

RISK FACTORS
- Family history of heart disease
- Family history of high lipid levels
- Atherosclerosis
- Hypertension
- Smoking
- Age (higher incidence in men over age 45 and women over age 55)
- Diabetes mellitus
- Sedentary lifestyle

AFTERCARE
- Encourage family members to take a cardiopulmonary resuscitation course (if appropriate).
- Tell the patient to seek help if the following occur:
  – chest pain
  – difficulty breathing.

HYPERTHYROIDISM

Hyperthyroidism results when the thyroid gland produces too much thyroid hormone. Causes include benign and malignant thyroid tumors, inflammation of the thyroid, and toxic nodular goiter. Grave's disease, the most common form of hyperthyroidism, results from an autoimmune response.

Because the thyroid gland regulates basic metabolism, the effects of increased metabolism appear throughout the body. Metabolic effects include weight loss (occasionally weight gain), heat intolerance, and low-grade fever. Cardiovascular effects include tachycardia, wide pulse pressure, systolic hypertension, and atrial fibrillation. Musculoskeletal effects include hand tremors and muscle weakness; GI effects include hepatomegaly and diarrhea; and endocrine effects include irregular menses, impotence, gynecomastia, decreased libido (delayed puberty in children), and infertility. The skin becomes dry and itchy, and the hair, thin and

TEACHING TOPICS

MEDICATIONS

- Beta blockers counteract the effects of thyroid hormone on the sympathetic nervous system.
- Thyroid hormone antagonists slow hormone production.
- Steroids reduce inflammation of tissue behind and around the eyes.
- Iodines increase the amount of thyroid hormone stored in the thyroid and reduce thyroid gland vascularity.
- Radioiodines irradiate and destroy thyroid cells, reducing thyroid hormone production.

ACTIVITY

- No overexertion (to avoid increasing body temperature)
- Maintaining a cool environment

NUTRITION

- High-calorie (4,000 to 5,000 calories/day), high-protein, high-carbohydrate diet (until patient reaches appropriate weight)
- Low-fiber diet (to minimize peristalsis)
- Low-salt diet for exophthalmic patient (to decrease swelling of tissues around the eyes)

fine. The disorder also results in such behavioral changes as constant fatigue, insomnia, anxiety, and irritability. Grave's disease causes striking exophthalmos, in many cases accompanied by conjunctivitis.

Although uncommon, life-threatening thyroid storm (thyrotoxicosis) can result from untreated hyperthyroidism. Such stressors as surgery, labor and delivery, infection, and myocardial infarction can also trigger this medical emergency.

POTENTIAL COMPLICATIONS
- Thyroid storm
- Arrhythmias
- Heart failure
- Shock
- Loss of vision
- Hypothyroidism (from treatment)

TREATMENTS
- Eye care for exophthalmos (wearing eye patches or sunglasses; avoiding dusty places; wearing a sleeping mask or taping eyes shut at night; raising the head of the bed to drain fluid; instilling artificial tears, eyedrops, or ointment)
- Relaxation techniques

RISK FACTORS
- Family history of hyperthyroidism
- Gender (higher incidence in women, particularly between ages 20 and 40)

AFTERCARE
- As appropriate, explain to the patient and family that the patient's hyperactive, irritable, unpredictable, and difficult behavior results from the disease.
- Tell the patient to weigh himself daily (at same time, on same scale, with same amount of clothing on), record weights, and report sudden or steady changes.
- Tell the female patient that pregnancy will be high risk.
- Tell the patient to seek help if the following occur:
  - tachycardia
  - vomiting
  - fever
  - blurred vision.

HYPOTHYROIDISM

Hypothyroidism results from insufficient production of thyroid hormone. Primary hypothyroidism, the most common type, is the loss of functional thyroid tissue, usually resulting from radioiodine treatment, thyroidectomy, or Hashimoto's disease. Secondary hypothyroidism is a rare condition that results from the pituitary gland's failure to produce thyroid-stimulating hormone.

Because the thyroid gland regulates basic metabolism, the effects of slowed metabolism appear throughout the body. Metabolic effects may include weight gain and cold intolerance; cardiovascular effects, a slowed heart rate, hyperlipidemia, and (sometimes) hypertension; musculoskeletal effects, muscle cramps and stiffness; and GI effects, decreased peristalsis and constipation. The patient feels lethargic and may become forgetful and depressed. He may become delusional or psychotic or may hallucinate, particularly if he's elderly. The skin becomes dry and bruises easily, the hair becomes dry and sparse, the nails thicken, the tongue swells, and the face grows coarse, puffy, and expressionless.

TEACHING TOPICS

MEDICATIONS

- Thyroid hormones (such as levothyroxine and liothyronine) supplement or replace hormones that the patient doesn't produce.

ACTIVITY

- Gentle exercise, as tolerated, with doctor's approval (patient may feel tired and unmotivated to try even low-level activity)

NUTRITION

- Low fat, low-cholesterol, low-calorie diet
- High-fiber diet

This thickening of the face and periorbital areas, called myxedema, is a hallmark of hypothyroidism and results from interstitial accumulation of mucin. It can occur in response to such stressors as illness and prolonged exposure to cold.

The thyroid gland may also increase in size as it tries to put out more thyroid hormone. Called a goiter, this enlarged thyroid can interfere with breathing and swallowing. Because the signs and symptoms of hypothyroidism typically develop slowly over months or years, the patient may not be diagnosed until he seeks treatment after a goiter develops.

Although uncommon, life-threatening myxedema coma can result from untreated hypothyroidism. Such stressors as surgery and infection can also trigger this medical emergency. Untreated hypothyroidism in children can result in mental and growth retardation. Treatment consists of thyroid-replacement therapy.

POTENTIAL COMPLICATIONS
- Myxedema coma
- Respiratory infection
- Heart failure

TREATMENTS
- Thyroid-replacement therapy
- Achieving and maintaining appropriate weight

RISK FACTORS
- Gender (higher incidence in women)
- Age (over age 50, but can be congenial)
- Family history of hypothyroidism
- Neck surgery
- Treatment for hyperthyroidism
- Certain medications (such as lithium, amiodarone, steroids, adrenergic agonists, phenytoin)

AFTERCARE
- Tell the patient to:
  – weigh himself daily (at same time, on same scale, with same amount of clothing on), record weights, and report sudden or steady changes
  – avoid abruptly stopping or changing thyroid replacement medications
  – avoid over-the-counter medications without the doctor's approval.
- Offer the patient and family on-going emotional support as needed.
- Tell the patient to seek help if the following occur:
  – increasing lethargy
  – weight gain
  – fever.

OBESITY

One of the most common health problems in the United States, obesity underlies many disorders, such as coronary artery disease, diabetes mellitus, and gout. A person weighing 20% or more above the appropriate weight for height and gender, as based on U.S. Department of Agriculture height and weight guidelines, is considered obese.

However, weight is only one way to evaluate obesity. Other ways include assessing the percentage of a patient's body fat (calculated by measuring subcutaneous skinfold thickness or by water displacement), calculating his body mass index (based on guidelines for appropriate body mass published by the National Institutes of Health), and determining his body frame. The distribution of fat also affects the risks obesity poses; fat in the upper-body area around the waist poses a greater risk than fat on the hips or thighs.

Because obesity results when energy intake exceeds energy output, treatment aims to counteract this imbalance, usually with diet and exercise. The main fac-

TEACHING TOPICS

MEDICATIONS

- Vitamin supplements (such as a daily multivitamin) supplement a very low-calorie diet.
- Appetite suppressants (such as diethylpropion, phentermine, phenylpropanolamine, and sibutramine) prevent hunger.

ACTIVITY

- Regular aerobic exercise (to increase metabolism and improve cardiovascular function)
- Short exercise sessions, gradually increased to 20- to 30-minute sessions at least three times a week
- Enjoyable, convenient activities (such as exercising with a friend or dog) to promote compliance

NUTRITION

- Restricted-calorie diet, with nutritional consult
- Maintaining a food diary, with notations about moods and feelings
- Planning meals and snacks throughout the day to prevent excessive hunger
- Taking cultural preferences and tastes into account in diet planning
- Understanding the importance of an appropriate breakfast
- Maintaining an appropriate caloric intake to achieve the desired weight loss (a deficit of 3,500 calories achieves the loss of 1 lb [0.45 kg] of fat)

tor in achieving and maintaining weight loss is the patient's motivation; he'll need much support and encouragement to lose weight and keep it from returning. Some patients may need appetite suppressants or surgery (such as gastric bypass or gastroplasty) to lose the necessary weight.

POTENTIAL COMPLICATIONS
- Diabetes mellitus
- Hypertension
- Atherosclerosis and heart disease
- Hypoventilation
- Gout
- Degenerative arthritis
- Back pain
- Sleep apnea
- Gallbladder disease

Treatments
- Stress management and relaxation techniques and behavior modification

Risk factors
- Family history of obesity
- Certain disorders (hypothyroidism, pituitary disorders)
- Inactivity

Aftercare
- As appropriate, suggest the patient join a support group or find a coach or mentor to help him lose weight.
- Tell the patient to seek help if the following occur:
  – chest pain
  – difficulty breathing
  – sudden, sharp abdominal pain
  – episode of fainting
  – depression.

BACK PAIN, LOWER

A common complaint, lower back pain refers to pain in the lumbar area. The pain can stem from any of the structures in this part of the back—bones, disks, facet joints, ligaments, muscles, or nerve roots. Pain that lasts over 6 months or recurs on a frequent or regular basis is considered chronic. Over 90% of the population of the United States will experience at least one episode of disabling back pain over the course of a lifetime.

Several conditions can cause lower back pain. Most cases result from activity or injury; chronic lower back pain commonly results from degenerative disk disease. Pain that radiates down the leg may signal nerve root involvement. Very rarely, back pain indicates systemic infection, aneurysm, or cancer.

TEACHING TOPICS

MEDICATIONS

- Narcotic analgesics (such as hydrocodone, oxycodone, propoxyphene, tramadol, and pentazocine) relieve pain (for short-term use only).
- Nonsteroidal anti-inflammatory drugs (such as acetaminophen and aspirin) reduce inflammation and relieve pain.
- Skeletal muscle relaxants (such as baclofen, carisoprodol, cyclobenzaprine, chlorzoxazone, and methocarbamol) help relax tight muscles, lessening pain.

ACTIVITY

- Bed rest for acute back pain (usually for not more than 48 hours)
- Regular exercise program (for general fitness and muscle strength, especially of abdominal muscles)
- No sitting for long periods (may aggravate pain)
- Participation in sports that avoid back stress (swimming, bicycling)
- No repetitive bending and twisting movements (can aggravate pain)

NUTRITION

- Reduced-calorie diet for the overweight patient

Treatment generally consists of pain medicine and muscle relaxants along with instruction in muscle-relaxation and pain-relief techniques. The patient's pain usually resolves within a few weeks. To prevent recurrence, the patient should learn how to modify activities to help prevent back injury. The patient with chronic back pain may also need to find ways to adapt his lifestyle to accommodate his limitations. That may mean that he can no longer sit for long periods, mow the lawn, or use heavy equipment such as a jackhammer. Such a patient also needs to learn good body mechanics. Some patients, such as those with degenerative scoliosis, may need surgical fusion to relieve pain.

POTENTIAL COMPLICATIONS
- Paresis from spinal cord compression
- Decreased mobility that interferes with activities of daily living

TREATMENTS
- Warm packs or heating pads (to improve circulation) and warm or ice packs (to reduce swelling, inflammation, muscle spasms, and pain)
- Good body mechanics
- Achieving and maintaining appropriate weight
- Transcutaneous electrical nerve stimulation (to relieve pain)
- Traction (to relieve muscle spasm)
- No tobacco use (increases the risk for chronic low back pain)
- Relaxation techniques and biofeedback
- Acupuncture (to reduce pain)

RISK FACTORS
- Poor body mechanics
- Poor posture
- Pregnancy
- Certain disorders (degenerative disk disease, spondylolisthesis, spinal stenosis, herniated disk, degenerative scoliosis)

AFTERCARE
- Tell the female patient that pregnancy places further strain on the back; recommend that she practice good body mechanics, rest, and use back and leg support when she lies down.
- Tell the patient to seek help if the following occur:
  – numbness and tingling of the legs
  – pain that radiates down one or both legs
  – weakness in one or both legs
  – loss of bowel or bladder control.

FIBROMYALGIA

Fibromyalgia is characterized by widespread soft-tissue pain, spasms, or both that can occur in 18 areas defined as tender points by the American College of Rheumatology. Affecting from 3 to 6 million people in the United States, mostly women, this poorly understood syndrome has only begun to receive recognition, study, and credibility within the past 10 years.

To be diagnosed with fibromyalgia, a patient must have pain on digital palpation of at least 11 of the 18 defined tender points, with a history of at least 3 months of widespread pain. Although it's not clear what causes the disorder, it seems to be related to abnormal central processing of pain sensations and possibly the loss of non-REM sleep. Secondary fibromyalgia may result from another rheumatic disorder, such as rheumatoid arthritis, systemic lupus erythematosus, or Sjögren's syndrome.

TEACHING TOPICS

MEDICATIONS

- Analgesics (such as short-term narcotics, non-steroidal anti-inflammatory drugs [only minimally helpful], and tramadol) lessen pain.
- Antidepressants (such as amitriptyline, doxepin, nortriptyline, and low-dose trazodone [taken at bedtime]) promote restorative sleep and help relieve pain.
- Skeletal muscle relaxants (such as baclofen, carisoprodol, chlorzoxazone, cyclobenzaprine, and methocarbamol) relax tightened muscles, easing pain and allowing more restful sleep.

ACTIVITY

- Warming up before exercising (helps prevent muscle strain and pain)
- Gentle stretching exercises (maintain muscle flexibility and reduce pain)
- Gentle aerobic exercise (maintains muscle strength and overall fitness)
- Water aerobics (maintain flexibility without aggravating pain); warm air temperature in pool and changing areas prevent chilling and muscle spasms
- Yoga (provides gentle stretching and exercise along with mental calming and relaxation)

NUTRITION

- Low-fat diet high in complex carbohydrates (may help some patients)
- No caffeine (may help some patients)

The patient with fibromyalgia typically experiences disrupted, unrefreshing sleep and may experience depression, anxiety, anger, or social withdrawal along with the pain. Other common symptoms include fatigue and morning stiffness. Disorders associated with fibromyalgia include migraine headaches, chronic fatigue syndrome, irritable bowel syndrome, and multiple drug allergies. The patient may suffer considerable emotional distress over the chronic nature of the pain and its effects on work and family life. The patient may also feel embarrassed by the skeptical reactions of others—including health care workers—to the vague and variable symptoms and lack of physical signs of the syndrome.

Treatment focuses on pain relief, exercise, and sleep. The patient may also need treatment for the depression, anger, and anxiety that may accompany the disorder.

POTENTIAL COMPLICATIONS

- Functional or emotional debilitation that interferes with activities of daily living

TREATMENTS

- Warm packs or heating pads (to improve circulation) and warm or ice packs (to reduce swelling, inflammation, muscle spasms, and pain)
- Transcutaneous electrical nerve stimulation (to relieve pain)
- Massage and acupuncture (during flare-ups)
- Stress management and relaxation techniques and biofeedback
- Improved coping skills and behavior modification methods

RISK FACTORS

- Rheumatic disorders (rheumatoid arthritis, systemic lupus erythematosus, Sjögren's syndrome)
- Gender (much higher incidence in women)
- Family history of similar pain and sleep patterns

AFTERCARE

- Offer emotional support and encouragement.
- Tell the patient:
  – to shift to and from daylight savings time in small increments over several days
  – who is a shift worker to consider switching to a job with steady hours to prevent sleep pattern disruption.
- Tell the patient to seek help if the following occur:
  – increased pain
  – coping mechanisms become inadequate
  – sleep pattern that doesn't improve or worsens.

FRACTURES

Defined as a break in a bone, a fracture typically results from such traumas as motor vehicle or work accidents, sports injuries, and falls. A patient who has weak bones—from osteoporosis or prolonged steroid therapy, for example—may suffer a pathologic fracture; stress fractures can result from repetitive use.

A fracture can be categorized in several ways. It's first categorized as open or compound (when the skin is broken) or closed. A fracture can also be classified by the pattern of the break (linear, oblique, longitudinal, transverse, or spiral), by the appearance of the fracture (burst, chip, complete, or displaced), by the type (avulsion, compression, comminuted, depressed, impacted, or overriding), and by the completeness of the break (greenstick).

Bleeding, bruising, edema, and inflammation of surrounding tissue; loss of function; crepitus; and pain—which can vary from tenderness to excruciating

TEACHING TOPICS

MEDICATIONS

- Nonnarcotic analgesics (such as acetaminophen and nonsteroidal anti-inflammatory drugs) help relieve pain.
- Narcotic analgesics (such as hydrocodone, oxycodone, propoxyphene, tramadol, and pentazocine) relieve pain that doesn't respond to nonnarcotic analgesics.
- Antibiotics (such as ceftriaxone, carbenicillin, and ticarcillin) combat infections from open fractures.

ACTIVITY

- Isometric and range-of-motion exercises as appropriate (help prevent stiffness and atrophy)
- Use of cane, crutches, or wheelchair as needed, with physical therapy consult for safe and correct use
- Weight bearing, as directed by the doctor (stimulates bone healing)

NUTRITION

- Adequate hydration and a high-fiber diet (to prevent constipation from decreased mobility)
- High-calcium, high-protein diet (to promote bone and tissue healing)
- Increased vitamin C and D intake (to promote bone healing)

pain—can all accompany a fracture. Although the fracture itself is rarely life-threatening, serious complications can arise. For example, muscle spasms can displace broken bones that can in turn damage blood vessels and nerves, or a fat embolism can enter the bloodstream and block an artery.

POTENTIAL COMPLICATIONS
- Shock
- Fat embolism
- Deep vein thrombosis and pulmonary embolism
- Artery and nerve damage
- Infection, gangrene, and necrosis of the bone
- Compartment syndrome
- Joint stiffness, immobility, deformity, or arthritis
- Reflex sympathetic dystrophy

TREATMENTS
- Closed or open reduction to restore displaced bone fragments to normal position with splinting or traction for immobilization
- Skin care (including pin care) for patient with external fixation device, traction, or cast
- Warm packs or heating pads (to improve circulation) and warm or ice packs (to reduce swelling, inflammation, muscle spasms, and pain)
- Comfort measures (such as talcum powder under cast to alleviate itching)

RISK FACTORS
- Osteoporosis
- Tobacco use (causes calcium to leach from bone)
- Trauma

AFTERCARE
- Teach the patient to:
  – keep his home well lighted, remove throw rugs, and take other measures to help prevent falls
  – check circulation and function in the affected extremity.
- Tell the patient to seek help if the following occur:
  – chest pain
  – difficulty breathing
  – fever
  – increase in pain
  – swelling
  – foul-smelling drainage
  – numbness and tingling
  – change in color and temperature of affected limb
  – loose pins on external fixation device.

HERNIATED DISK

Normally, intervertebral disks—made up of cartilage surrounding the soft, gelatinous nucleus pulposus—separate and cushion the vertebrae in the spinal column. However, when injury or straining force the nucleus pulposus through a fragile portion of the cartilage (particularly likely if the disk has already degenerated), a herniated disk results. The herniated disk (also called a slipped or ruptured disk or a herniated nucleus pulposus) then compresses spinal nerve roots, resulting in irritation (radiculopathy) and back pain.

Herniation typically occurs in the lumbar area, particularly between L4 and L5. It can also occur in the cervical area and, rarely, the thoracic area. Causes in younger patients include direct injury to the spine and strenuous physical activity,

Teaching topics

Medications

- Narcotic analgesics (such as codeine, hydromorphone, meperidine, morphine, and propoxyphene) relieve pain (for short-term use only).
- Skeletal muscle relaxants (such as baclofen, carisoprodol, cyclobenzaprine, chlorzoxazone, and methocarbamol) help relax tight muscles, lessening pain.
- Nonsteroidal anti-inflammatory drugs (such as ibuprofen and naproxen) relieve pain.

Activity

- Bed rest on a firm mattress
- Body positioning and back-strengthening exercises, with physical therapy consult
- Lying down when sitting becomes uncomfortable
- Logrolling to change positions when lying down
- Alternating activity with rest to prevent overexertion
- No sitting for long periods (may aggravate back pain); keeping feet propped and knees higher than hips when sitting
- Energy-conservation measures and equipment, with occupational therapy consult

Nutrition

- High-fiber diet (to prevent constipation from inactivity and narcotic analgesic use)
- Adequate fluid intake (to prevent constipation)
- Reduced-calorie diet for the overweight patient

such as heavy lifting. In older patients, degeneration of disk cartilage can lead to herniation.

The main symptom is severe pain that radiates down the extremity innervated by the compressed nerve root. For instance, if herniation occurs in the lumbar area, compression of the sciatic nerve leads to pain that follows the course of the nerve across the hip and down the buttocks and leg. The patient may also experience numbness or tingling and muscle spasms or weakness in the extremity. Movement, coughing, and laughing worsen the pain; rest relieves it.

POTENTIAL COMPLICATIONS
- Paralysis or paresis (from nerve compression)
- Sciatica

TREATMENTS
- Warm packs or heating pads or ice packs
- Good body mechanics
- Maintaining appropriate weight
- Transcutaneous electrical nerve stimulation
- Back brace, support, or a cervical collar (to provide support until muscle strength returns)
- Traction (to relieve muscle spasm)
- Laminectomy
- Spinal fusion
- Microdiskectomy
- Chemonucleolysis (injection of chymopapain into herniated disk to dissolve the nucleus pulposus)

RISK FACTORS
- Heavy lifting with poor body mechanics
- Gender (higher incidence in men)
- Back injury

AFTERCARE
- Offer the patient emotional support; recovery may take months (up to a year) and pain may become chronic.
- Tell the patient to seek help if the following occur:
  – increased pain
  – development of or increase in numbness or weakness
  – loss of movement in the affected extremity.

MUSCULAR DYSTROPHY

Muscular dystrophy (MD) is a group of inherited disorders characterized by progressive degeneration of skeletal muscle. Defects in the genes that control muscle function result in muscle weakness, the hallmark of these disorders. Several theories attempt to explain how this weakness results. One suggests a problem in the nerve-muscle connection; another points to insufficient blood flow to the muscles as the cause. One of the more promising theories suggests that defective cell membranes in the muscles allow proteins and enzymes to leak out, resulting in wasting of the muscle fibers; connective and fatty tissue then replace these wasted fibers.

Several types of MD occur. The most common type, Duchenne's MD only occurs in boys; it generally strikes during early childhood and results in death by the early 20s. Other types include Becker's MD, Emery-Dreifuss MD, facioscapulohumeral MD, and oculopharyngeal MD. Patients with the less degenerative types of MD may have normal life expectancies.

TEACHING TOPICS

MEDICATIONS

- Steroids (such as prednisone) provide short-term improvement in muscle strength.

ACTIVITY

- Gentle, regular exercise as tolerated; alternating exercise with rest to prevent overexertion
- Swimming and water aerobics (prevents stress on joints)
- Passive stretching, without forcing joints past the point of resistance (delays and minimizes contractures)
- Energy-conservation measures and equipment, with occupational therapy consult

NUTRITION

- High-fiber diet (to prevent constipation from inactivity)
- Adequate hydration (to prevent constipation)

A delay in walking may lead to the diagnosis of Duchenne's MD at around 18 to 24 months, although some children aren't diagnosed until they reach school-age, when the abnormal gait becomes obvious. A child with Duchenne's MD typically walks on his toes and appears to waddle, with his abdomen pushed forward, and demonstrates Gower's maneuver. The disorder may impair intellectual ability in some children, although others may do well in school. Many patients must use a wheelchair by adolescence, and patients commonly develop scoliosis and contractures. Scoliosis and weak respiratory muscles can lead to respiratory infections and breathing difficulty, which can result in respiratory failure—a common cause of death in Duchenne's MD.

POTENTIAL COMPLICATIONS
- Respiratory failure
- Heart failure
- Fractures

TREATMENTS
- Achieving and maintaining appropriate weight
- Back support, body jacket, or braces for patient with scoliosis
- Full length, weight-bearing orthopedic devices as needed
- Splints, braces, and wheelchair as needed
- Deep-breathing exercises and postural drainage (to prevent respiratory complications)
- Relaxation techniques and biofeedback
- Smoking cessation and avoiding secondhand smoke
- Assisted breathing at night as needed (with intermittent positive-pressure ventilation, a rocking bed, or a body shell)

RISK FACTORS
- Family history of MD
- Gender (higher incidence in males)

AFTERCARE
- Tell the patient (or caregiver if appropriate) that the patient should:
  – wear medical identification
  – receive an annual flu vaccination.
- Explain that gene therapy shows promise for future treatment.
- Offer the patient and the family emotional support and (if needed) counseling.
- Recommend genetic counseling (if appropriate).
- Tell the patient or caregiver to seek help if the following occur:
  – difficulty breathing
  – difficulty swallowing.

OSTEOARTHRITIS

Previously, osteoarthritis was thought to result from the normal wear and tear on joints that occurs during aging. More recently, researchers have come to believe that various factors play a role in the development of osteoarthritis, including cartilage metabolism, inflammatory responses, and genetics. Primary (idiopathic) osteoarthritis develops during aging and appears to have a genetic predisposition. Secondary osteoarthritis can stem from repetitive joint overuse (which damages cartilage), injury, disorders such as gout and septic arthritis, and medications such as colchicine. The disorder strikes more than 60 million Americans, and most people over age 45 have osteoarthritic changes in hip and knee joints.

The hallmark of osteoarthritis is degeneration and loss of cartilage in the joint spaces. As the cartilage breaks down, bony spurs may form and deposits of cartilage and bone debris appear in the joint space, resulting in inflammation and swelling. Joints affected include the hips and knees (both weight-bearing joints),

TEACHING TOPICS

MEDICATIONS

- Analgesics (such as acetaminophen, propoxyphene, and tramadol) reduce pain.
- Topical analgesics (such as triethanolamine and capsaicin) applied over painful joints provide pain relief.
- Nonsteroidal anti-inflammatory drugs (such as aspirin, salsalate, choline magnesium trisalicylate, magnesium salicylate, sulindac, nabumetone, and etodolac) decrease inflammation and pain.

ACTIVITY

- Exercise as tolerated; alternating exercise with rest to avoid overexertion
- Range-of-motion and isometric exercises
- Energy-conservation measures and equipment, with occupational therapy consult
- Use of cane or crutches as needed, with physical therapy consult for safe and correct use
- Swimming and water aerobics (prevents stress on joints)
- Planned rest regimen for patient receiving intra-articular steroid injections

NUTRITION

- Healthy diet based on recommended portions from the food pyramid

the spine, the distal interphalangeal joints (where Heberden's nodes appear), and the base of the thumb. Initially, the patient may feel just a dull ache in the affected joint. As the disease progresses, he may have chronic pain, stiffness, and swelling from bone enlargement and may lose mobility and function.

Treatment is generally conservative and includes resting the affected joint, using splints, and controlling pain with medication and heat. Patients with more disabling disease may require intra-articular steroid injections, joint lavage, or arthroscopy. Surgical options include osteotomy, bone fusion, and joint replacement. Research into gene modification holds promise, and drugs to prevent cartilage degeneration and to improve viscosity and lubrication in the joint spaces are in development. Some of these drugs are already in use outside the United States.

POTENTIAL COMPLICATIONS
- Loss of function in an extremity
- Deformity of one or more joints

TREATMENTS
- Splints, back support, or braces (to support and rest joints)
- Warm packs or heating pads (to improve circulation) and warm or ice packs (to reduce swelling, inflammation, muscle spasms, and pain)
- Transcutaneous electrical nerve stimulation (to relieve pain)
- Relaxation techniques, biofeedback, ultrasound, distraction, and imagery (to relieve pain)
- Achieving and maintaining appropriate weight

RISK FACTORS
- Family history of osteoarthritis
- Gender (higher incidence in women, especially postmenopausal women)
- Age (adults over age 75)
- Obesity
- Trauma
- Repetitive overuse of joints

AFTERCARE
- If appropriate, remind the patient that osteoarthritis usually isn't a crippling disease and that measures (including surgery) are available to help manage pain and promote function.
- Tell the patient to seek help if the following occur:
  – increased pain
  – decreased joint mobility.

OSTEOPOROSIS

Osteoporosis results when bone mass decreases (the result of a greater rate of bone resorption than formation), leaving bones brittle. Patients with osteoporosis are at increased risk for fractures, not only from trauma but also from normal activities, such as sitting down, reaching, and bending. These pathological fractures typically occur in the pelvis, vertebra (eventually resulting in shorter stature and kyphosis), and radius. The disorder primarily affects the elderly.

Primary osteoporosis can result from menopause in women (type I) and from aging in both men and women (type II). Secondary osteoporosis results from another disorder or medication. Contributing factors to osteoporosis include a low peak bone mass (the maximum bone density achieved during the lifetime, which is genetically influenced) and menopause, which causes a drop in estrogen that

TEACHING TOPICS

MEDICATIONS

- Calcium supplements help replace calcium and prevent bone resorption.
- Vitamin D supplements help the body absorb and use calcium.
- Estrogen replacements help maintain bone mass.
- Calcium regulators slow bone resorption.
- Calcium-regulating hormones block bone resorption.
- Analgesics help relieve pain from fractures.

ACTIVITY

- Weight-bearing exercises as tolerated (to slow resorption)
- Bed rest, as ordered, for fractures
- Water aerobics (as a transition back to weight-bearing exercise)
- Physical therapy consult before exercising for patients with kyphosis or pain
- Modification of exercise program or supplemental calcium for women with exercise-induced amenorrhea

NUTRITION

- 1,000 to 1,500 mg per day of calcium for postmenopausal woman
- High-calcium diet, with nutritional consult
- No excessive sodium or caffeine intake
- Limited alcohol intake, as ordered by doctor

leads to a rapid loss of bone mass. The patient may not be diagnosed with the disorder until he seeks treatment for a pathological fracture.

Preventive measures include adequate calcium intake and weight-bearing exercise (to slow the resorption of bone). However, regular dietary intake may not provide enough calcium to achieve a high peak bone mass, particularly in girls. Treatment for existing osteoporosis aims to arrest the development of the disease with calcium supplements and, when possible, with appropriate weight-bearing exercises.

POTENTIAL COMPLICATIONS
- Skeletal fractures and complications from fractures
- Inability to breathe adequately because of kyphosis

TREATMENTS
- Use of supports and corsets during activities (to relieve pain)
- Warm packs or heating pads (to improve circulation) and warm or ice packs (to reduce swelling, inflammation, muscle spasms, and pain)
- Transcutaneous electrical nerve stimulation or ultrasound (to relieve pain)
- Relaxation techniques, biofeedback, distraction, and imagery (to relieve pain)
- Smoking cessation

RISK FACTORS
- Gender
- Race
- Body frame
- Family history of osteoporosis
- Not bearing children
- Sedentary lifestyle
- Immobility
- Certain disorders (rheumatoid arthritis, hyperthyroidism, liver disease, chronic obstructive pulmonary disease)
- Certain medications (steroids, methotrexate, heparin, phenytoin, isoniazid)
- Heavy smoking
- Heavy alcohol consumption
- Insufficient calcium intake

AFTERCARE
- Tell the patient:
  – to keep his home well lighted, use handrails, remove throw rugs, and take other measures to help prevent falls
  – taking estrogen replacements to receive annual gynecologic and breast examinations
  – taking vitamin D supplements to have calcium levels checked regularly.
- Tell the patient to seek help if the following occur:
  – difficulty breathing
  – increase in pain
  – swelling or stiffness that persists after a fall.

SPRAINS AND STRAINS

Typically caused by hyperextension, a sprain is damage to ligament, the fibrous tissue that joins the articular ends of bones and stabilizes joints. A strain is an injury to a tendon—the fibrous tissue that attaches skeletal muscle to bone—or to muscle. Strains result from overextending muscles or tendons. An acute strain can result from stretching a muscle or tendon too far (during exercise, for example); a chronic strain results from regular overuse.

These injuries can be categorized by degree. First-degree describes a minor tearing or stretching of the fibers, with some discomfort but without bruising, swelling, or loss of range of motion. A second-degree sprain or strain involves partial (up to 80%) tearing, with muscle spasms, swelling, pain, later bruising, and some loss of range of motion. A third-degree sprain or strain is a complete rupture or tearing, with muscle spasms, swelling, bruising, severe pain, and loss of function. A patient with a third-degree sprain or strain typically feels a tearing, popping, or burning sensation at the site of the injury; he may need surgery to repair the injury.

Treatment typically follows the RICE protocol:

- *Rest*, to prevent the injury from becoming worse, can last from a day or two to a couple of months.

TEACHING TOPICS

MEDICATIONS

- Nonsteroidal anti-inflammatory drugs (such as ibuprofen, naproxen, and aspirin) help decrease inflammation and relieve pain.

ACTIVITY

- Use of crutches as needed, with a physical therapy consult for safe use

NUTRITION

- Healthy diet based on recommended portions from the food pyramid

- *Ice* reduces inflammation and swelling and relieves muscle spasms, bruising, and pain. The patient can place ice over the tender area (in a plastic bag or towel, never directly on the skin) for 20 to 30 minutes at a time every couple of hours while awake for the first 48 hours after the injury. After that, the patient can switch to gentle heat, which can soothe the injury and promote the reabsorption of blood.
- *Compression* with a snug—but not too tight—elastic bandage helps decrease bleeding, swelling, and pain.
- *Elevation* of the affected part above the level of the heart minimizes swelling and prevents venous pooling.

POTENTIAL COMPLICATIONS
- Nerve damage
- Loss of function of affected part
- Joint instability

TREATMENTS

- Splint, back support, or brace (to support and rest injured joint)
- Warm packs or heating pads (to improve circulation) and warm or ice packs (to reduce swelling, inflammation, muscle spasms, and pain)
- Transcutaneous electrical nerve stimulation or ultrasound (to relieve pain)

RISK FACTORS

- Not warming up before sports activity
- Continuing to use a painful joint

AFTERCARE

- Tell the patient that using the injured area too soon after injury can worsen the injury or result in reinjury.
- Tell the patient to seek help if the following occur:
  – decreased range of motion
  – change in color or temperature of affected part.

TENDINITIS AND BURSITIS

Contrary to what the name implies, tendinitis isn't inflammation of a tendon; it's inflammation of the fluid-filled synovial sheath that surrounds and protects certain tendons from rubbing directly against a bone. Common types of tendinitis include thoracic outlet syndrome, tennis elbow, and carpal tunnel syndrome (which affects 2 million people in the United States each year). Bursitis is inflammation of one or more bursae—small synovial fluid-filled pouches that provide cushioning between bony structures. Bursae are found throughout the body, mostly in joints and between tendons and bones, although a few pad spaces between bone and skin. Bursitis can occur in shoulders, elbows, hips, heels, and especially knees (housemaid's knee).

Tendinitis and bursitis typically result from repetitive movement that results in irritation—for instance, from certain types of jobs (window washing, painting,

TEACHING TOPICS

MEDICATIONS

- Steroids (such as triamcinolone, prednisolone, betamethasone, methylprednisolone, and dexamethasone injected into the tendon sheath or bursa) reduce inflammation and pain.
- NSAIDs (such as indomethacin, ibuprofen, ketoprofen, naproxen, and nabumetone) reduce inflammation and pain.

ACTIVITY

- Stopping, changing, or modifying the pain-producing activity
- Use of braces, cane, or crutches, as needed
- Stretching and muscle-strengthening exercise to prevent recurrence

NUTRITION

- Healthy diet based on recommended portions from the food pyramid

dentistry, typing) and some sports (tennis, golf, bowling). Some anatomic malformations, such as scoliosis and unequal leg length, and certain diseases, such as gout and rheumatoid arthritis, can also cause tendinitis or bursitis.

Treatment for either type of inflammation starts with rest, reducing the aggravating activity, and possibly immobilizing the affected part. Treatment may also include splinting, hot and cold packs, gentle stretching exercises, nonsteroidal anti-inflammatory drugs (NSAIDs), and (if necessary) injection of steroids into the inflamed sheath or bursa. Follow-up treatment may include gentle remobilization exercises and possibly modifying or stopping the aggravating activity.

POTENTIAL COMPLICATIONS
- Joint immobility

TREATMENTS
- Warm packs or heating pads (to improve circulation) and warm or ice packs (to reduce swelling, inflammation, muscle spasms, and pain)
- Elevation of swollen, painful extremities
- Possible use of orthotics, such as splints, braces, or slings (to immobilize the joint)

RISK FACTORS
- Sports that involve frequent repetitive movements (tennis, golf)
- Repetitive movements (meat cutting, typing, window washing)

AFTERCARE
- If the patient uses a computer regularly, teach him about ergonomically correct positioning.
- If the patient needs a cane, teach him how to use it.
- Tell the patient to seek help if the following occur:
  – increasing pain and swelling
  – increasing loss of function of affected part.

BENIGN PROSTATIC HYPERPLASIA

Affecting 50% of men by age 60 and 90% of men by age 85, benign prostatic hyperplasia (BPH) is noncancerous enlargement of the prostate gland. This enlargement stems from an increase in the number of cells. As the prostate grows larger, it compresses the urethra, resulting in increased resistance to urine flow. It also reduces bladder space, resulting in urinary frequency and urgency and nocturia. Although the cause of the disorder isn't known, it seems to develop only in the presence of testicular androgens. The disorder rarely causes serious health complications, but it can interfere with day-to-day life.

TEACHING TOPICS

MEDICATIONS

- 5-alpha reductase inhibitors (such as finasteride) lower prostate-specific antigen levels and reduce the size of prostatic tissue, allowing an increase in urine flow.
- Adrenergic blocking agents (such as doxazosin and terazosin) relax the smooth muscle of the prostate and bladder neck, improving voiding.

ACTIVITY

- As tolerated

NUTRITION

- Adequate fluid intake (to prevent urinary infection and calculi formation)
- No alcohol (because of its diuretic effects)

Signs and symptoms develop slowly. The patient may gradually notice an increase in urinary frequency, hesitancy in starting the stream of urine, a decrease in the force of the stream, and sometimes blood in the urine. Urge incontinence occurs in some patients.

POTENTIAL COMPLICATIONS
- Impaired urination
- Azotemia
- Urine retention, possibly leading to infection or calculi
- Renal insufficiency

TREATMENTS
- Possibly an indwelling urinary or intermittent catheter (to relieve urine retention)
- Warm sitz baths
- Voiding whenever the urge is felt
- Surgical procedures include:
  – transurethral needle ablation, microwave therapy, or balloon dilation of the prostate
  – insertion of a uretheral stent
  – transurethral ultrasound guided laser incision of prostate and ultrasound high-intensity prostate ablation
  – transurethral incision or resection
  – prostatectomy.

RISK FACTORS
- Age (men over age 50)

AFTERCARE
- Tell the patient:
  – to have an annual prostate examination to detect BPH after age 40
  – who is impotent after surgery to receive sexual counseling (as appropriate)
  – to avoid sympathomimetic drugs because they aggravate the symptoms of BPH
  – taking an adrenergic blocking agent that he may initially experience postural hypotension
  – not to decrease fluid intake to avoid urgency and frequency; instead, suggest spacing fluids throughout the day and not drinking too much at one time.
- Tell the patient to seek help if the following occur:
  – increasing difficulty voiding
  – fever and chills
  – cloudy, foul-smelling urine
  – pain when voiding.

GLOMERULONEPHRITIS

Glomerulonephritis refers to a group of diseases that affects the glomeruli. In glomerulonephritis, antigen-antibody complexes—part of the body's immune response to infection—lodge in the glomeruli, causing inflammation. A secondary immune response results in increased permeability of the basement membranes of the glomeruli. The disease can develop in association with such disorders as systemic lupus erythematosus, systemic vasculitis, amyloidosis, Goodpasture's syndrome, and Schönlein-Henoch purpura.

The disease can occur in an acute, chronic, or rapidly progressive form. The most common acute form is poststreptococcal glomerulonephritis and typically develops in children and young adults 2 to 3 weeks after a streptococcal infection of the throat or skin. Infectious glomerulonephritis develops during or within a couple of days of a bacterial, viral, or parasitic infection.

TEACHING TOPICS

MEDICATIONS

- Antibiotics (such as penicillin) combat the initial infection.
- Immunosuppressants (such as azathioprine and cyclosporine) inhibit the immune response.
- Steroids (such as prednisone) decrease inflammation and promote tissue healing.
- Antihypertensives (such as enalapril and captopril) normalize blood pressure.
- Diuretics (such as furosemide, bumetanide, hydrochlorothiazide, and metolazone) stimulate the production of urine.
- Antilipemics (such as pravastatin and lovastatin) decrease lipid levels.

ACTIVITY

- Bed rest for the patient with acute glomerulonephritis (initially); gradual return to usual activities
- Alternating activity with rest to prevent overexertion
- Regular aerobic exercise (to help manage hyperlipidemia)
- No prolonged sitting with feet dependent (to prevent peripheral edema)
- Periodic ankle range-of-motion exercises (to promote circulation)

NUTRITION

- High-calorie diet
- Low-sodium, low-potassium diet
- Use of ice, lip moisturizers, and other ways to maintain restricted fluid intake
- Possibly protein-restricted diet, based on glomerular filtration rate, with nutritional consult for renal diet

In chronic glomerulonephritis, an inflammatory process destroys the glomeruli, and the kidneys become fibrous and shrunken. The patient may feel vaguely unwell for years before renal insufficiency becomes obvious. If end-stage renal disease develops, the patient will need dialysis or kidney transplantation.

A devastating form of the glomerulonephritis, rapidly progressive glomerulonephritis results in the destruction of many of the glomeruli over a few weeks. The patient may experience hypertension, produce little or no urine, and develop hematuria, edema, abdominal pain, and acidosis.

POTENTIAL COMPLICATIONS
- End-stage renal disease
- Heart failure

TREATMENTS
- Measuring and recording intake and output
- Blood pressure monitoring
- Support hose for patient with peripheral edema
- Smoking cessation
- Skin care for edematous areas
- Hemodialysis or peritoneal dialysis for azotemia, intractable acidosis, hyperkalemia that doesn't respond to other therapies, or diuretic-resistant pulmonary edema

RISK FACTORS
- Bacterial, viral, and parasitic infections
- Certain disorders (systemic lupus erythematosus, systemic vasculitis, amyloidosis, Goodpasture's syndrome, Schönlein-Henoch purpura)

AFTERCARE
- Tell the patient to:
  – weigh himself daily, record weights, and report sudden or steady changes
  – avoid over-the-counter medications that contain sodium or aspirin.
- Tell the sexually active female patient to use contraception to avoid pregnancy but not to use oral contraceptives while taking antibiotics.
- Tell the patient to seek help if the following occur:
  – weight increase of more than 2 lb (0.9 kg) in 1 day
  – urine output under 600 ml in 1 day
  – fever
  – blood pressure outside parameters set by the doctor.

PYELONEPHRITIS

Pyelonephritis is an inflammation of the renal pelvis that results from bacterial infection. The most common causative agent is *Escherichia coli*, although other gram-negative and (rarely) gram-positive bacteria can also cause the disorder. The bacteria typically invade the renal pelvis through the ascending route, making their way up the urinary tract from the perineum. Occasionally, an infection elsewhere in the body—even on the skin—causes pyelonephritis, although this usually happens only in immunocompromised or chronically ill patients. Bacteria can also spread through the lymphatic system, although this occurs rarely.

A patient with pyelonephritis may not have painful, frequent urination and urgency—the classic signs and symptoms of a urinary tract infection. The patient may instead experience high fever, chills, flank pain, body aches, and possibly nausea, vomiting, and diarrhea. He may also have cloudy, foul-smelling urine.

TEACHING TOPICS

MEDICATIONS

- Antibiotics (such as ciprofloxacin, ofloxacin, and trimethoprim-sulfamethoxazole) combat the infection.
- Narcotic or nonnarcotic analgesics relieve pain.

ACTIVITY

- As tolerated

NUTRITION

- Additional fluid intake (to flush kidneys)
- No alcohol or caffeine during antibiotic treatment and course of the disease

Most patients recover quickly with antibiotic treatment. However, some patients may have recurrences and develop chronic disease. These patients may have scarring and shrinking of the kidneys, with resulting renal failure.

POTENTIAL COMPLICATIONS
- Sepsis
- Renal abscess or necrosis
- Hydronephrosis
- Renal scarring
- Acute renal failure
- Emphysematous pyelonephritis (in patients with diabetes mellitus)

TREATMENTS
- Smoking cessation

RISK FACTORS
- Gender (higher incidence in women)
- Pregnancy
- Diabetes mellitus
- Hypertension
- Infection with human immunodeficiency virus
- Neurogenic bladder
- Recurring renal calculi
- Recurring bladder infections
- Prostatic infection
- Indwelling or intermittent catheterization
- Abnormal urinary tract

AFTERCARE
- Tell the female patient to:
  – clean her perineum from front to back after urination
  – stop using oral contraceptives (if applicable) and use another contraceptive while taking antibiotics (antibiotics can prevent oral contraceptives from working).
- Tell the patient:
  – to avoid bath salts and bubbles, which can irritate the perineum
  – with recurring pyelonephritis to take showers rather than tub baths.
- Tell the patient to seek help if the following occur:
  – persistent fever and chills
  – flank pain
  – worsening pain.

RENAL CALCULI

Renal calculi are deposits that form in the urinary tract by crystallizing around a nucleus of precipitated material. They may consist of calcium (most common), oxalate, cystine, uric acid, or a combination of these materials; struvite calculi, another type of renal calculi, result when magnesium and ammonium phosphate crystallize around a bacterial nucleus.

Most renal calculi form in the kidneys and either lodge there or move down the urinary tract, where they can pass out of the body or become lodged in the urinary tract. Most calculi pass without surgical intervention.

TEACHING TOPICS

MEDICATIONS

- Narcotic analgesics (such as codeine, hydromorphone, and oxycodone) help relieve renal colic.
- Urinary analgesics and antispasmodics (such as phenazopyridine, flavoxate, and propantheline) relieve pain and spasms of the urinary tract.
- Medications specific to the composition of calculi or underlying disorder help treat those disorders.

ACTIVITY

- As tolerated

NUTRITION

- Low-calcium, low-oxalate, or low-purine diet (based on the composition of the calculi)
- Extra fluids (to flush the urinary tract and help pass calculi)

The patient typically seeks treatment for the severe renal or ureteral pain associated with passing calculi, the hallmark symptom of renal calculi. The patient may also have blood or puss in his urine. Some patients may experience only mild pain, and a few pass renal calculi with no pain.

POTENTIAL COMPLICATIONS
- Urinary tract obstruction
- Renal infection
- Hydronephrosis
- Renal insufficiency

TREATMENTS
- Possible collection of a 24-hour urine specimen
- Extracorporeal shock wave lithotripsy
- Percutaneous nephrolithotomy
- Nephrectomy (as a last resort if other treatments are not successful)

RISK FACTORS
- Gender (higher incidence in men, especially those ages 20 to 40)
- Location (higher incidence in the southeastern United States)
- Family history of renal calculi
- Dehydration
- Urinary tract infection
- Certain medications (acetazolamide, calcium carbonate, sodium bicarbonate, aluminum hydroxide)
- Sedentary lifestyle

AFTERCARE
- Strain the patient's urine to obtain calculi for analysis.
- Tell the patient to seek help if the following occur:
  – increase in pain
  – fever
  – cloudy or foul-smelling urine
  – inability to void
  – appearance or continuation of blood in urine.

RENAL FAILURE, ACUTE

Acute renal failure (ARF) results from abrupt failure of the kidneys (over hours to days) to excrete waste products and to balance fluids and electrolytes. Such a failure results in a buildup of nitrogenous wastes, fluid and electrolyte imbalance, and inadequate urination. The condition commonly signals an underlying disorder, typically a cardiovascular disorder.

ARF is usually categorized as prerenal, intrinsic, or postrenal. It can also be classified as oliguric (excretion of less than 400 ml/day of urine) or nonoliguric; the prognosis is worse with the oliguric form.

Prerenal failure stems from conditions that reduce blood flow to the kidneys. Such causes include hemorrhage, vomiting, diarrhea, and diuretic use. Conditions that reduce cardiac output, conditions that decrease peripheral vascular resistance, conditions that block blood flow to the kidneys, and a dissecting aneurysm can also cause prerenal failure.

Intrinsic failure stems from damage to the kidneys, usually from glomerulonephritis or acute tubular necrosis. Nephrotoxic drugs, such as aminoglyco-

TEACHING TOPICS

MEDICATIONS

- Diuretics (such as furosemide and mannitol) stimulate urine production, although their use is controversial.
- Laxatives (such as sorbitol) help eliminate potassium in stools.
- Medications specific to the underlying cause of ARF help treat those disorders.

ACTIVITY

- Possible bed rest or very limited activity (to conserve energy)

NUTRITION

- High-calorie, low–complete-protein diet
- Diet low in sodium, potassium, and phosphorus
- Fluids restricted to volume of urine output plus 500 ml daily
- Use of ice, lip moisturizers, and other ways to maintain restricted fluid intake

sides, amphotericin B, and contrast media, can also trigger intrinsic failure, as can trauma to the kidney.

Postrenal failure results from obstruction of any part of the urinary tract. Causes include renal calculi, tumors, prostatic hyperplasia, blood clots, retroperitoneal fibrosis, neurogenic bladder, and strictures or stenosis of the ureters or urethra.

Early signs of ARF include weight gain, edema, and decreased urine output. Other signs and symptoms depend on the cause of the failure and may include chest pain, hematuria, and difficult and painful urination.

POTENTIAL COMPLICATIONS
- Secondary infections
- Pericarditis
- Seizures
- Anemia
- Stress ulcers

TREATMENTS
- Accurate measuring of fluid intake and urine output
- Blood pressure monitoring
- Hydration and salt-loading
- Meticulous electrolyte monitoring to detect hyperkalemia
- Dialysis (if the patient becomes hyperkalemic)
- Daily weight

RISK FACTORS
- Reduced blood flow to kidneys (from bleeding, severe vomiting, diarrhea)
- Primary glomerulonephritis
- Ureter, urethra, or bladder neck obstruction
- Certain disorders (hypertension, systemic lupus erythematosus, coronary artery disease)
- Chronic renal failure
- Certain nephrotoxic medications (aminoglycosides, amphotericin B, contrast media)

AFTERCARE
- Tell the patient to weigh himself daily (at same time, on same scale, with same amount of clothing on), record weights, and report sudden or steady changes.
- Tell the patient to seek help if the following occur:
  – sudden drop in urine output
  – fever
  – shortness of breath
  – difficulty breathing
  – chest pain.

RENAL FAILURE, CHRONIC

Chronic renal failure (CRF) describes a progressive, irreversible condition in which damaged and destroyed nephrons eventually leave the kidneys unable to excrete waste products and regulate fluid and electrolyte balance. Causes include hypertension and other systemic disorders, although the cause in a specific case may not be clear.

In the first stage of CRF, the patient may have reduced renal reserve but no symptoms. Renal insufficiency follows, with such signs and symptoms as anemia, dehydration, increased output of dilute urine, and possibly nocturia. As the disease progresses, renal failure results in electrolyte imbalances. End-stage renal disease involves all body systems, resulting in decreased urine output; dry, itchy, orange-colored skin; appetite loss; nausea and vomiting; difficulty breathing; osteomala-

TEACHING TOPICS

MEDICATIONS

- Angiotensin-converting enzyme inhibitors (such as captopril) reduce blood pressure.
- Erythropoietin (such as epoetin alfa) raises red blood cell production and corrects the anemia associated with CRF.
- Vitamin K supplements (such as calcitriol) prevent calcium loss from bone.
- Calcium supplements (such as calcium carbonate and aluminum hydroxide) prevent calcium loss from bone.

ACTIVITY

- Regular aerobic exercise (to prevent calcium loss from the bone and maintain muscle strength)
- Alternating activity with rest to prevent overexertion

NUTRITION

- Protein-restricted diet, with nutritional consult
- Phosphate restriction (dairy products, cola soft drinks)
- Low-potassium diet with low-phosphorus bran (to help prevent constipation)
- Water intake limited to maintain sodium concentration of 135 to 145 mEq/L
- Vitamin supplements

cia; osteoporosis; restless leg syndrome; peripheral edema; lethargy; impaired cognitive function; depression; personality changes; and possibly psychosis.

When the patient reaches end-stage renal disease, the only treatment options include hemodialysis or peritoneal dialysis and kidney transplant.

POTENTIAL COMPLICATIONS
- Uremia
- Hypertension
- Anemia
- Hyperkalemia
- Bone disease
- Coronary artery disease
- Cardiac complications (heart failure, pericarditis, tamponade)

TREATMENTS
- Hemodialysis or peritoneal dialysis (continuous ambulatory, automated, continuous cyclic, intermittent, nightly)
- Shunt care for the patient on hemodialysis
- Extra emphasis on oral hygiene, regular dental care, and skin care (using moisturizing soaps and lotions)
- Treatment of underlying cause

RISK FACTORS
- Diabetes mellitus
- Glomerulonephritis
- Hypertensive renal or cystic disease
- Race (higher incidence in Native Americans and blacks)
- Cigarette smoking

AFTERCARE
- Offer the patient and family support; arrange for counseling and social services consults as appropriate.
- Tell the patient:
  – to tell all doctors, dentists, and health care professionals that he has CRF
  – to avoid over-the-counter medications without the doctor's approval
  – that sexual dysfunction may occur
  – on hemodialysis how to care for his shunt.
- Tell the patient to seek help if the following occur:
  – sudden decrease or absence of urine output
  – sudden weight gain
  – swelling of feet and ankles
  – fever
  – trouble breathing.

URINARY INCONTINENCE

The involuntary loss of urine, urinary incontinence affects many women, particularly those over age 60. Men experience this disorder much less frequently than women, typically after prostatectomy.

Urinary incontinence can result from various causes. Acute incontinence may be an adverse effect of certain medications, occur during a urinary tract infection, or result from anxiety.

Forms of chronic incontinence include stress, urge, overflow, reflex, and functional. The most common type, stress incontinence occurs when a sudden increase in intra-abdominal pressure—from lifting, laughing, sneezing, coughing, or another stress—forces a small amount of urine past a weak urinary sphincter. Hyperreflexia, or spasms, of the detrusor muscle can cause urge incontinence, in which the patient feels the urge to urinate but can't hold back the flow long

TEACHING TOPICS

MEDICATIONS

- Alpha- and beta-adrenergic antagonists promote smooth-muscle contraction at the bladder outlet.
- Antispasmodics relax the detrusor muscles, increasing bladder capacity and decreasing the urge to void.
- Anticholinergic agents relax the detrusor muscle.
- Cholinergics (such as bethanechol) increase detrusor tone, promoting more complete bladder emptying.
- Estrogen replacements help improve pelvic muscle tone, improving control of urination.
- Periurethral collagen injections may increase urethral tone.

ACTIVITY

- Maintaining voiding diary (including time, presence or absence of urge, instances of incontinence and activity [laughing, lifting], and amount of urine voided)
- Using techniques to initiate voiding at scheduled voiding times (running water, pouring warm water over the perineum)
- Using adult diapers as needed during activities (allows mobility and provides skin protection)

NUTRITION

- Adequate hydration (to stimulate micturition and prevent infection and renal calculi formation)
- No caffeine, carbonated drinks, alcohol, or spicy foods (as appropriate)
- Timing fluid intake so the patient can stay dry during the night (as appropriate)

enough to reach a bathroom. In overflow incontinence, the patient may not feel any urge to urinate despite an overextended bladder. Exertion or activity may precipitate the overflow, which occurs without contraction of the detrusor muscle. A patient with reflex incontinence—the result of spinal cord injury and such disorders as spina bifida—has no voluntary bladder control. Functional incontinence can occur when the patient is immobile, can't find or reach a bathroom, or can't undress in time.

POTENTIAL COMPLICATIONS
- Urinary tract infections
- Pyelonephritis
- Infection and septic shock
- Skin erosion

TREATMENTS
- Intermittent or indwelling catheterization
- External catheterization (for men)
- Kegel exercises
- Bladder training
- Vaginal cone, pessary, or ring (to provide bladder neck support or strengthen pelvic muscles)
- Use of electrical stimulation device
- Surgical options (rare) include artificial urinary sphincter and use of internal slings
- Biofeedback
- Achieving and maintaining appropriate weight

RISK FACTORS
- Gender (higher incidence in women, especially in elderly women)
- Certain medications (diuretics, sedatives, cardiac drugs)
- Urinary tract infection
- Neurologic factors (dementia, cerebrovascular accident, spinal cord injury, neurogenic bladder)

AFTERCARE
- Teach the patient about treatments and aids to help combat embarrassment, depression, and social withdrawal.
- Tell the patient to seek help if the following occur:
- cloudy, discolored, or foul-smelling urine
- fever
- chills
- flank pain
- inability to void.

URINARY TRACT INFECTION

Urinary tract infections (UTIs) result when the urinary tract becomes infected with one of several bacteria. Causative organisms include *Escherichia coli, Klebsiella, Enterobacter, Pseudomonas,* and *Staphylococcus.*

Women are far more susceptible to UTIs than men, in part because of a shorter urethra and the proximity of the anus to the urethra. However, male infants under a year have a higher incidence of UTIs than do female infants, probably because of congenital abnormalities. UTIs in adult males are typically associated with kidney or prostate infection and commonly result from antibiotic-resistant organisms.

TEACHING TOPICS

MEDICATIONS

- Antibiotics (such as amoxicillin, ciprofloxacin, norfloxacin, and cefaclor) eradicate the bacteria responsible for the infection.
- Bacteriostatic agents (such as trimethoprim, sulfisoxazole, sulfamethoxazole, and nitrofurantoin) inactivate bacteria.
- Urinary analgesics and antispasmodics (such as phenazopyridine, flavoxate, and propantheline) relieve pain and spasms of the urinary tract.

ACTIVITY

- As tolerated
- No bicycling or horseback riding (may worsen the infection)
- Voiding after sexual intercourse (flushes bacteria from the urinary tract)
- No sexual intercourse when symptoms are present

NUTRITION

- Intake of at least 3 qt (3 L) of water per day
- Increased intake of acidic foods (meats, eggs, cheese, such fruits as cranberries, prunes, and plums)

UTIs can affect the lower urinary tract, involving the bladder and urethra (cystitis), or the upper urinary tract, involving the kidney and its pelvis (pyelonephritis). Cystitis occurs more commonly, but pyelonephritis poses a greater risk because it endangers kidney function. Signs and symptoms of cystitis include burning pain during urination; low back pain; urinary frequency and urgency; voiding of small amounts of urine; cloudy, foul-smelling urine; and the feeling that the bladder hasn't fully emptied. The patient may also experience fever, chills, nausea and vomiting, and flank pain. Treatment consists of fluids and medication to combat the infection.

POTENTIAL COMPLICATION
- Pyelonephritis

TREATMENTS
- Bladder irrigation with amphotericin B (for a patient with an indwelling catheter)
- Suppression therapy for recurrent cystitis (taking small doses of nitrofurantoin or trimethoprim at regular intervals)

RISK FACTORS
- Gender (much higher incidence in women)
- Sexual activity
- Pregnancy
- Wearing synthetic underwear and tight pants
- Indwelling urinary catheterization, particularly long-term use
- Neurogenic bladder
- Benign prostatic hyperplasia

AFTERCARE
- Tell the female patient to:
  – wipe from front to back after urination
  – avoid tight underwear and pants
  – avoid bath salts and bubbles, which can irritate the perineum
  – take showers rather than tub baths if she's prone to cystitis
  – stop using oral contraceptives (if applicable) and use another contraceptive while taking antibiotics.
- Tell the patient to seek help if the following occur:
  – pain and burning that don't clear up within one or two days
  – persistent fever and chills
  – flank pain.

EPISTAXIS

Rarely a serious disorder, epistaxis (nosebleed) results from disruption of the nasal mucosa. Drying of or picking at the mucosa is the most common cause. Trauma, such as a blow to the face, is the second most common cause and can result in sudden, forceful bleeding. A chronic trickle of serosanguinous fluid may signal nasal or sinus cancer. Epistaxis can also result from a coagulation disorder.

Bleeding typically occurs from vessels along the nasal septum, which has only a thin mucosal layer. The most common site is Kiesselbach's area, located on the anterior septum and richly supplied with blood. Although less common, bleeding from the posterior septum may result in more severe bleeding because the area contains larger blood vessels than does the anterior septum.

TEACHING TOPICS

MEDICATIONS

- Systemic antibiotics prevent toxic shock syndrome and sinusitis in patients with posterior nasal packing.
- Topical vasoconstrictors decrease bleeding.
- Local anesthetics decrease discomfort.

ACTIVITY

- Sitting down and leaning forward during bleeding; no lying down
- No nose blowing for several hours
- Sports and activities with minimal risk of trauma to the face and nose (if bleeding is recurrent)

NUTRITION

- Adequate fluids (to compensate for blood loss)
- Healthy diet based on recommended portions of the food pyramid

Most occurrences are managed on the spot with manual compression and possibly ice. If these measures don't control bleeding within 10 to 15 minutes, the patient needs further treatment to prevent significant blood loss. Anterior nasal packing soaked in a vasoconstrictor and local anesthetic is usually the next step. Other treatments include cauterization of the site with silver nitrate or electrocautery and balloon compression. A patient with posterior bleeding may need anterior-posterior tamponade; if bleeding continues, he may require surgical arterial ligation.

POTENTIAL COMPLICATIONS
- Blood loss
- Shock
- Aspiration of blood

TREATMENTS
- Pinching the nose shut for 5 to 10 minutes when bleeding starts
- Digital pressure on the forehead or upper lip
- Ice pack on the nose during bleeding
- Nasal packing or balloon systems
- Cool mist humidifier (for patient with nasal packing and during winter to prevent nasal drying)

RISK FACTORS
- Irritation, injury, or infection of the nose
- Nasal tumors
- Breathing dry, heated air
- Family history of recurrent nosebleeds
- Certain diseases (atherosclerosis, hypertension, Hodgkin's disease, leukemia, telangiectasia, hemophilia and other coagulation disorders)
- Certain medications (anticoagulants [most often aspirin], antineoplastics)
- Cocaine snorting

AFTERCARE
- Tell the sexually active female patient to stop using oral contraceptives (if applicable) and to use another contraceptive while taking antibiotics (antibiotics can prevent oral contraceptives from working).
- Tell the patient to seek help if the following occur:
  – bleeding that isn't controlled in 10 to 15 minutes
  – recurrent epistaxis.

GLAUCOMA

One of the leading causes of blindness in the United States, glaucoma is characterized by an increase in pressure within the eye. This pressure decreases the blood supply to the optic nerve, eventually leading to irreversible vision loss and blindness. In almost all cases, the increased intraocular pressure results when an obstruction prevents the drainage of aqueous humor — which is constantly being produced — from the anterior chamber of the eye.

Chronic open-angle glaucoma, the most common form of the disorder, causes no symptoms in the early stages. When detected at this early stage (typically during a regular eye examination by a pressure check), treatment can generally prevent vision loss and blindness. By the time such symptoms as blurred peripheral vision and halos appear, damage has already occurred.

TEACHING TOPICS

MEDICATIONS

- Beta blockers (such as betaxolol and timolol) decrease intraocular pressure by reducing the secretion of aqueous humor.
- Sympathomimetic drugs (such as epinephrine and dipivefrin) decrease intraocular pressure by promoting the drainage of aqueous humor.
- Miotics (such as pilocarpine and carbachol) improve the drainage of aqueous humor.
- Carbonic anhydrase inhibitors (such as acetazolamide, dichlorphenamide, and methazolamide) decrease the production of aqueous humor.
- Prostaglandins (such as latanoprost) increase the outflow of aqueous humor.

ACTIVITY

- No straining at stool or lifting heavy objects (increases intraocular pressure)

NUTRITION

- High-fiber diet and adequate, but not excessive, fluids (to help prevent constipation)

Primary angle-closure glaucoma, an emergency situation, results from the abrupt and complete obstruction of the outflow of aqueous humor. Intraocular pressure rises to dangerous levels within just a few hours. Signs and symptoms include pain, redness, blurred vision, rainbow-colored halos, headache, and sometimes nausea and vomiting.

Primary developmental glaucoma occurs in infants, and secondary glaucoma may result from an injury to the eye, an eye tumor, or certain systemic diseases, such as diabetes and hypertension.

POTENTIAL COMPLICATIONS
- Visual impairment and blindness

TREATMENTS
- Prescribed eyedrops and ointments
- Argon laser trabeculoplasty or trabeculectomy, if drug treatment is ineffective

RISK FACTORS
- Certain diseases (diabetes mellitus, hypertension)
- Myopia
- Family history of glaucoma
- Eye injury
- Age (higher incidence in elderly people)
- Race (higher incidence in African Americans)

AFTERCARE
- Teach the patient how to administer eyedrops or ointment:
  – close eye and press on inner corner for 1 to 3 minutes.
- Tell the patient:
  – to keep his home well lighted, not to use throw rugs, and to take other measures to help prevent falls
  – not to use unprescribed eye medication.
- Suggest that family members over age 35 be tested for glaucoma.
- Tell the patient to seek help if the following occur:
  – severe eye pain
  – vision changes (blurring, photophobia, seeing halos or rainbows)
  – tearing
  – headache
  – nausea or vomiting.

LARYNGITIS

Laryngitis is an inflammation of the voice box, or larynx. One of the most common causes of laryngitis is overuse of the voice by excessive yelling, singing, or shouting. The coughing, throat clearing, purulent drainage, and mouth breathing associated with a cold also commonly cause this disorder. Gastroesophageal reflux disease (GERD) can result in laryngitis when reflux of gastric acid burns the larynx; it can take several weeks for laryngeal tissue to heal. Other causes include allergies, exposure to irritants, and (occasionally) emotional or psychiatric problems.

Hoarseness, the key symptom of laryngitis, occurs when the vocal cords become inflamed and swollen. The patient needs more expiratory effort to move air

TEACHING TOPICS

MEDICATIONS

- Cough suppressants suppress a nonproductive cough, preventing further throat irritation.
- Gastric acid inhibitors decrease acid production in GERD.
- Gastrointestinal stimulants promote rapid emptying of the stomach in GERD.
- Antibiotics destroy bacteria in sinusitis.
- Sympathomimetics provide nasal decongestion and reduce laryngeal swelling.
- Antihistamines decrease inflammation in allergies.
- Steroids can provide short-term reduction of inflammation.

ACTIVITY

- No whispering (can strain the inflamed larynx); using note writing for communication
- No strenuous throat clearing (worsens inflammation)
- Alternating activity with rest to prevent overexertion

NUTRITION

- Dietary modifications for patients with GERD
- Adequate water intake (to thin mucus in the throat and allow laryngeal healing)

across the swollen cords, making the voice strained and rough. The patient may also experience pain on swallowing or speaking.

Treatment consists of resting the voice, eliminating causative factors, and providing optimal conditions for laryngeal healing. Laryngitis usually resolves within one or two weeks. Laryngitis that lasts longer than 2 weeks may indicate a more serious conditions, such as laryngeal cancer or, in children, papilloma.

POTENTIAL COMPLICATIONS
- Airway obstruction
- Permanent voice impairment

TREATMENTS

- Resting the voice
- Cool mist humidifier use
- Hot showers (steam may relieve throat symptoms)
- Gargling with warm, salty water (may relieve throat symptoms)
- Elevating head of bed (to prevent reflux in patients with GERD)
- Smoking cessation and avoiding second-hand smoke
- Throat lozenges or hard candy (to help keep the throat lubricated)

RISK FACTORS

- GERD
- Smoking
- Endotracheal intubation
- Emotional or psychiatric problems
- Exposure to inhaled irritants (smoke, dust, chemical fumes)
- Certain disorders (rheumatoid arthritis, hypothyroidism)

AFTERCARE

- Tell the sexually active female patient to stop using oral contraceptives (if applicable) and to use another contraceptive while taking antibiotics (antibiotics can prevent oral contraceptives from working).
- Tell the patient to seek help if the following occur:
  – symptoms last over 2 weeks
  – fever
  – difficulty breathing
  – inability to swallow liquids
  – coughing that produces blood-tinged sputum.

PHARYNGITIS

Pharyngitis is an inflammation or infection of the pharynx that causes a sore throat. Common causes include viral and bacterial infections; less common causes include allergies, irritants, trauma, and cancer. Hand washing, proper disposal of used tissues, and avoiding close contact during the illness can help prevent its spread.

Viral infections account for most cases of pharyngitis, typically from an adenovirus or a rhinovirus. Influenza and herpes viruses can also cause the disorder. Besides the hallmark sore and scratchy throat, signs and symptoms may include conjunctivitis, a runny nose, coughing, hoarseness, mouth lesions, and diarrhea.

Several types of bacteria can cause pharyngitis, including group C, G, and F streptococci and *Neisseria gonorrhoeae*. However, infection with group A beta-

TEACHING TOPICS

MEDICATIONS

- Antibiotics (such as penicillin, amoxicillin, erythromycin, azithromycin, and cephalexin) combat the causative organism in bacterial pharyngitis.
- Steroids (such as prednisone) decrease inflammation and swelling.
- Local analgesics (such as lidocaine [Viscous Xylocaine]) can numb the throat if swallowing becomes painful.

ACTIVITY

- As tolerated; no overexertion
- No contact sports if the patient has mononucleosis (may result in injury to the enlarged spleen)

NUTRITION

- Adequate water intake (to thin mucus in the throat and prevent dehydration)
- Soft or liquid diet (may be better tolerated while the throat is very sore)
- Dietary modifications for patients with gastroesophageal reflux disease (GERD)

hemolytic streptococci (GABHS) poses the greatest risk because the patient may develop acute rheumatic fever with possible heart valve damage, acute glomerulonephritis from antigen-antibody complexes lodging in the glomeruli, and toxic shock syndrome. Signs and symptoms of pharyngitis caused by GABHS include the sudden onset of sore throat with pain on swallowing; fever, possibly accompanied by headache; a rash; swollen lymph nodes under the jaw; nausea and vomiting; and abdominal pain.

POTENTIAL COMPLICATIONS
- Airway obstruction (from a swollen pharynx)
- Acute rheumatic fever (from GABHS)
- Acute glomerulonephritis (from GABHS)
- Toxic shock syndrome (from GABHS)

TREATMENTS
- Cool mist humidifier use
- Hot showers (steam may relieve throat symptoms)
- Gargling with warm, salty water (may relieve throat symptoms)
- Elevating head of bed (to prevent reflux in patients with GERD)
- Smoking cessation and avoiding secondhand smoke

RISK FACTORS
- GERD
- Smoking
- Endotracheal intubation
- Allergies
- Mononucleosis
- Exposure to inhaled irritants (smoke, dust, chemical fumes)
- Age (higher incidence of GABHS in children ages 5 to 15)

AFTERCARE
- If the patient is a child, tell his parents not to give him aspirin because of the risk of developing Reye's syndrome.
- Tell the sexually active female patient to stop using oral contraceptives (if applicable) and to use another contraceptive while taking antibiotics (antibiotics can prevent oral contraceptives from working).
- Tell the patient to seek help if the following occur:
  – difficulty breathing
  – blood in the urine
  – sudden drop in urine output.

SINUSITIS

Sinusitis is the inflammation of the membranes lining the paranasal sinuses. This inflammation increases secretions and causes the membranes to swell. The swelling, in turn, can prevent normal drainage, leaving the sinuses filled with mucus and pus — a perfect environment for bacterial or viral growth. Sinusitis most commonly occurs in the maxillary sinus, followed by the ethmoid and frontal sinuses and, less commonly, the sphenoid sinuses, located near the ears. Infection can also occur in all four sinuses simultaneously.

Sinusitis can be acute or chronic. *Streptococcus pneumoniae* and *Haemophilus influenzae* are most often at fault in acute sinusitis. Chronic sinusitis typically follows a persistent bacterial infection. Acute sinusitis causes a sharp or stab-

Teaching topics

Medications

- Antibiotics (such as amoxicillin, cefuroxime, cefpodoxime, loracarbef, cefaclor, and amoxicillin-clavulanate) combat the bacteria causing the infection.
- Decongestants (such as pseudoephedrine and phenylephrine) cause vasoconstriction of sinus membranes, relieving congestion.
- Nasal steroid sprays (such as fluticasone, beclomethasone, triamcinolone, budesonide, and flunisolide) decrease inflammation and congestion.
- Analgesics relieve pain.

Activity

- As tolerated; no overexertion

Nutrition

- Adequate water intake (to thin mucus and prevent dehydration)

bing pain and tenderness around the affected sinus, which worsens in the morning and when the patient bends over or coughs. Headache, fever, fatigue, pharyngitis, postnasal drainage, and a purulent nasal discharge also occur. Chronic sinusitis typically causes milder, less specific symptoms, including some loss of the sense of smell.

If antibiotics and decongestants don't clear sinusitis, the patient may need sinus irrigation or possibly surgery to drain the sinuses.

POTENTIAL COMPLICATIONS
- Meningitis
- Epidural, subdural, or brain abscess
- Eye infection (especially in children)

TREATMENTS
- Cool mist humidifier use
- Hot showers (steam may relieve congestion)
- Warm, moist compresses over the face (may be soothing)
- Smoking cessation, avoiding secondhand smoke, and avoiding exposure to inhaled irritants such as dust
- Nasal window procedure, Caldwell-LUC procedure, ethmoidectomy, and elastoplastic flap

RISK FACTORS
- Abnormalities of the ostia and surrounding area
- Septal deviation
- Immunodeficiency
- Secretion disorders (cystic fibrosis)
- Allergic rhinitis
- Upper respiratory infections
- Nasal blockage (from a nasogastric or nasotracheal tube or nasal packing)

AFTERCARE
- Tell the patient not to use over-the-counter nasal sprays or drops (they may interact with prescribed medications).
- Tell the sexually active female patient to stop using oral contraceptives (if applicable) and to use another contraceptive while taking antibiotics (antibiotics can prevent oral contraceptives from working).
- Tell the patient to seek help if the following occur:
  – fever and chills
  – edema of the eyelids.

TINNITUS

A symptom rather than a disease, tinnitus is intermittent or constant ringing, tinkling, jingling, or buzzing sounds that patients hear in one or both ears. Most patients aren't too bothered by it, but some patients find it unbearable. Tinnitus can also signal an underlying disorder. Causes can range from excessive cerumen or disturbances of hair cells in the inner ear to acoustic tumors.

Objective tinnitus — sounds that others beside the patient can hear — can result from several causes. The turbulent flow of blood can cause arterial and venous noises, and the stapedius, tensor tympani, and palatal muscles can produce clicking, banging, or popping sounds. The more common type, subjective tinni-

TEACHING TOPICS

MEDICATIONS

- Antidepressants (such as amitriptyline and nortriptyline) given at bedtime help the patient tolerate the sounds.
- Anesthetics (such as tocainide and mexiletine) may help decrease tinnitus.
- Anticonvulsants (such as carbamazepine, phenytoin, and primidone) may decrease tinnitus.
- Diuretics (such as hydrochlorothiazide) may decrease tinnitus in Ménière's disease.

ACTIVITY

- As tolerated; no activities that exacerbate sounds
- Alternating activity with rest to avoid fatigue (fatigue seems to worsen sounds)

NUTRITION

- Healthy diet based on recommended portions of the food pyramid
- No caffeine (may decrease tinnitus in some patients)

tus produces sounds that only the patient can hear. Most patients with tinnitus also have some hearing loss.

Unless an underlying cause can be found and treated, no cure for tinnitus exists. Some medications and other treatments can lessen symptoms for some patients. A patient may have to try several methods to find a treatment or combination of treatments that works best for him.

POTENTIAL COMPLICATIONS
- Anxiety or depression (from sounds)

Treatments

- Hearing aid (to improve hearing and allow normal sounds to mask the tinnitus)
- White-noise generator, fan, or air conditioner (to mask tinnitus)
- Tinnitus instrument (combination hearing aid and masker)
- Auditory habituation (training the patient to ignore the tinnitus)
- Stress management and relaxation techniques and biofeedback

Risk factors

- Excessive cerumen (ear wax)
- Chronic otitis externa or media
- Otosclerosis
- Certain medications (quinine)
- Age (higher incidence in elderly people)
- Acoustic tumors
- Ménière's disease

Aftercare

- Reassure the patient that most patients with tinnitus, even those who have some hearing loss, don't become deaf.
- Tell the patient to seek help if the following occur:
  – diminished hearing acuity
  – worsening tinnitus.

VERTIGO

In vertigo, the patient feels as if the environment is moving or spinning around him or that he is spinning around. This symptom can result from disorders of the semicircular canals, vestibular labyrinth, or inner ear. All of these disorders affect the sense of balance, which is normally maintained by the complex interaction of the vestibular system, the eyes, the proprioceptive sensors in the joints and muscles, and the cerebellum.

Several types of vertigo exist. In motion sickness — one of the most common types — the patient's eyes report a stationary environment and the vestibular system reports movement. As a result, the patient feels nauseous and unwell and may experience excessive salivation, yawning, and vomiting.

Benign positional vertigo occurs when a person gets into or out of bed or lifts his head up after bending over. It results from tiny bits of debris in the posterior semicircular canal (the result of injury or aging).

TEACHING TOPICS

MEDICATIONS

- Sedatives (such as diazepam and droperidol) help manage acute vertigo and nystagmus.
- Antiemetics (such as prochlorperazine, metoclopramide, and promethazine) control nausea and vomiting.
- Antivertiginous agents (such as meclizine) decrease vertigo without sedation.

ACTIVITY

- Bed rest (initially), possibly in a darkened room; slow movements, with minimal head movement
- Balance exercises when appropriate (to speed rehabilitation)

NUTRITION

- Adequate fluid intake if the patient is vomiting (to prevent dehydration)

Acute vertigo with nystagmus, nausea, and vomiting can result from an infection or lesion that causes an imbalance in the vestibular pathways. Recurrent attacks may occur with certain conditions, such as autoimmune diseases of the ear, Ménière's disease, transient ischemic attacks, labyrinthitis secondary to syphilis, and migraine headaches. Treatment of the underlying disease usually prevents the return of acute vertigo. Chronic vertigo can result in a permanent loss of vestibular function, although it usually results in milder, periodic attacks.

POTENTIAL COMPLICATIONS
- Injuries from falls
- Anxiety about future attacks
- Depression from the interruption of activities of daily living

TREATMENTS
- Vertigo rehabilitation, with physical therapy consult

RISK FACTORS
- Ménière's disease
- Labyrinthitis

AFTERCARE
- Tell the patient:
  – that he shouldn't drive until the cause has been successfully treated or he has undergone vertigo rehabilitation
  – to keep his home well lighted, not to use throw rugs, and to take other measures to help prevent falls.
- Tell the patient to seek help if the following occur:
  – worsening vertigo
  – loss of effectiveness of medication
  – persistent vomiting or dehydration
  – injury from a fall.

ATOPIC DERMATITIS

Atopic dermatitis is a chronic, noninfectious, inflammatory skin disorder associated with a personal or family history of asthma, hay fever, or allergic rhinitis. It seems to be related to the body's inability to modify the immunoglobulin E antibody response to antigens. The disorder is marked by acute flare-ups, which then subside for a time. Flare-ups and exacerbations of the condition can result from exposure to dust mites, some foods, stress, menstruation, dry skin, certain fabrics, and chemicals. The condition generally improves in the summer, perhaps because of exposure to sunlight and higher humidity.

Onset usually starts before age 5, typically on the face and extremities. Many children outgrow the disorder by adulthood. Although rare, adult onset is possi-

TEACHING TOPICS

MEDICATIONS

- Systemic or topical steroids (such as prednisone for short-term use, triamcinolone acetonide, and hydrocortisone) relieve itching and inflammation.
- Systemic antibiotics (such as erythromycin and dicloxacillin) combat bacterial infection.
- Antihistamines (such as hydroxyzine, doxepin, and cetirizine) relieve itching.
- Topical keratolytics (such as coal tar and anthralin) reduce inflammation.
- Systemic biological response modulators (such as gamma interferon and thymopoietin) reduce the frequency and severity of infections.

ACTIVITY

- Identifying and avoiding triggers
- Limiting activities that cause sweating during flare-ups (sweating aggravates dermatitis)
- No sudden changes in temperature and humidity

NUTRITION

- No foods (typically milk and eggs) that trigger a reaction

ble; when it occurs, the disorder is severe and persistent, affecting mostly the neck and the antecubital and popliteal areas.

Itching, one of the main symptoms, often affects the eyelids. If the patient doesn't receive treatment, scratching may introduce a secondary infection, a common occurrence. A patient with an acute inflammation develops red, edematous skin with crusty papules and plaques. Repeated flare-ups can lead to thickened, hardened skin with fissures and cracks, possibly with alopecia and changes in pigmentation.

POTENTIAL COMPLICATIONS
- Secondary bacterial, viral, and fungal infections

TREATMENTS
- Soaks with tar preparations followed by application of occlusive dressings
- Maintaining a cool, only moderately humid environment
- 100% cotton clothing when possible; no woolen, tight, or rough clothes
- Smoking cessation and avoiding secondhand smoke
- Minimizing dust, pollution, and animal dander
- Tar shampoo
- Mild, nonperfumed soap
- Emollients and topical steroids applied while body is damp after bathing
- Cold packs
- Stress management

RISK FACTORS
- Personal or family history of asthma, allergic rhinitis, hay fever, or food allergies
- Emotional stress
- Gender (slightly higher incidence in men)
- Age (usually develops in childhood)

AFTERCARE
- Tell the patient to:
  – read food labels to avoid foods that trigger a reaction
  – receive regular eye examinations (ocular complications can occur).
- Tell the sexually active female patient to stop using oral contraceptives (if applicable) and to use another contraceptive while taking antibiotics (antibiotics can prevent oral contraceptives from working).
- Tell the patient to seek help if the following occur:
  – fever
  – chills
  – drainage from lesions.

CONTACT DERMATITIS

A common disorder, contact dermatitis is an inflammation of the skin that results from direct contact with an irritating substance. It can occur as irritant or allergic and may be acute, subacute, or chronic.

Irritant contact dermatitis typically results from contact with a chemical or toxin. Some of the more common irritants include household and industrial cleaners, detergents, fuels, lubricants, metals (such as nickel and zinc), and jellyfish stings. In the acute stage, the area of contact becomes red, swollen, scaly, and itchy and develops lesions and blisters. If the disorder becomes chronic, the skin may thicken and fissure and the dermatitis may spread beyond the area of contact.

Allergic contact dermatitis develops only after a patient has become sensitized to a substance. Common allergens include certain plants (such as poison ivy,

TEACHING TOPICS

MEDICATIONS

- Antihistamines (such as diphenhydramine, hydroxyzine, cetirizine, loratadine, astemizole, and fexofenadine) reduce inflammation and itching.
- Systemic steroids (such as prednisone) and topical steroids (such as hydrocortisone, desonide, desoximetasone, and augmented betamethasone) reduce inflammation and itching.
- Systemic antibiotics (such as penicillin, erythromycin, tetracycline, and cephalosporins) and topical antibiotics (such as mupirocin) combat bacterial infection.
- Antipruritics (such as calamine lotion) soothe the skin and reduce itching.

ACTIVITY

- Identifying and avoiding irritants or allergens
- Wearing gloves, long sleeves, and other protective gear for activities where contact may occur

NUTRITION

- No foods that trigger a reaction

oak, and sumac), nut oil, some foods, and some hair-care products. In the acute stage, the area of contact becomes severely itchy, red, and swollen, with papules, plaques, and vesicles; the irritation may also spread to other parts of the body. Chronic inflammation may result in dry, thickened, cracked skin.

Patch testing can determine the substance responsible for the dermatitis. The patient should then avoid the substance or use protective clothing and barrier creams to protect the skin. The patient may need topical steroids for an acute reaction or short-term treatment with systemic steroids; the patient with chronic dermatitis shouldn't receive long-term steroid treatment.

POTENTIAL COMPLICATIONS
- Exfoliative dermatitis

TREATMENTS
- Moisturizing, nonperfumed soaps
- Cool compresses
- Compresses with Burow's solution
- Oatmeal baths
- Moisturizing or emollient lotions, creams, and ointments
- Barrier creams that contain polyamine salt and linoleic acid dimers

RISK FACTORS
- Occupation that requires contact with common allergens (health care workers, bricklayers, beauticians)

AFTERCARE
- If appropriate, suggest allergen patch testing.
- Tell the sexually active female patient to stop using oral contraceptives (if applicable) and to use another contraceptive while taking antibiotics (antibiotics can prevent oral contraceptives from working).
- Tell the patient to seek help if the dermatitis spreads or worsens.

DERMATOPHYTOSIS AND CANDIDIASIS

Fungal skin infections are common in the United States. Two of the most prevalent are dermatophytosis and candidiasis.

Also called *tinea*, dermatophytosis can take many forms: *tinea corporis* is found on the face, neck, and extremities; *tinea cruris* (jock itch) infects the groin and inner thighs; *tinea capitis* (ringworm) affects the scalp; *tinea pedis* (athlete's foot) infects the feet; and *tinea unguium* affects the fingernails and toenails. The infection typically looks like a ring, with a central clear area, although some patients have just a slight scaling.

Candida albicans exists normally in the GI and vaginal tracts of humans. However, predisposing factors — such as diabetes mellitus, obesity, decreased im-

TEACHING TOPICS

MEDICATIONS

- Topical antifungals treat local candidiasis and dermatophytosis.
- Antifungal powders treat tinea pedis and tinea unguium.
- Antiseborrheic agents control itching and flaking of the scalp and reduce the spread of infectious spores in tinea capitis.
- Antibacterials are used to wash the scalp and reduce the spread of infectious spores in tinea capitis.
- Systemic antifungals treat systemic candidiasis, urinary tract candidiasis, extensive or resistant dermatophytosis and, rarely, local candidiasis.

ACTIVITY

- Regular aerobic exercise

NUTRITION

- Healthy diet based on recommended portions of the food pyramid

munity, and use of antibiotics, systemic steroids, or oral contraceptives — may allow the organism to proliferate. It grows well in such moist environments as the mouth (thrush) and the vagina as well as in skin folds (intertrigo), particularly in people who sweat a great deal, such as laborers and athletes. Typically, the affected areas become red, raw, and itchy. In intertrigo, pustules and plaques may develop around the edges of the affected areas.

Many patients use over-the-counter medications to treat dermatophytosis and candidiasis. Because it can spread so quickly through school, tinea capitis is of particular concern. Affected children and their families must receive treatment before the children can return to school.

POTENTIAL COMPLICATIONS
- Alopecia

TREATMENTS
- Keeping skin cool and dry

RISK FACTORS
- Age (higher incidence of tinea capitis in children; higher incidence of candidiasis in infants and children)

Candidiasis
- Jobs or activities that lead to frequent, heavy sweating
- Trauma
- Moisture
- Obesity
- Diabetes mellitus
- Immunosuppression
- Certain medications (oral contraceptives, systemic antibiotics, steroids)

AFTERCARE
- Tell the patient taking itraconazole not to take astemizole (Hismanal) or cisapride (Propulsid).
- Tell the sexually active female patient to stop using oral contraceptives (if applicable) and to use another contraceptive while taking antibiotics (antibiotics can prevent oral contraceptives from working).
- Tell the patient to seek help if signs and symptoms of secondary infection occur.

HERPES SIMPLEX AND HERPES ZOSTER

Several types of herpes viruses affect humans, including herpes simplex and herpes zoster. Herpes simplex virus 1 (HSV-1) causes cold sores; herpes simplex virus 2 (HSV-2), genital herpes; and varicella-zoster virus (VZV), chickenpox and shingles.

Most of the cold sores that develop on the lips or mouth arise from HSV-1 infection; HSV-2 causes most cases of genital herpes. An outbreak of either type starts with tingling and burning. The area then becomes red and blistered. Ulcers form, crust over, and finally heal in about 2 weeks. Stress appears to trigger an outbreak. HSV-1 spreads through oral contact, and HSV-2 is sexually transmitted. Genital herpes in a pregnant woman can result in birth defects or the death of the baby.

TEACHING TOPICS

MEDICATIONS

- Systemic and topical antivirals (such as acyclovir, famciclovir, and valacyclovir) prevent the outbreak of or speed the healing of HSV and VZV lesions.
- Antidepressants (such as amitriptyline and carbamazepine) help reduce pain in PHN.
- Systemic steroids (such as prednisone) reduce inflammation in PHN.
- Topical analgesics (such as capsaicin and lidocaine) decrease pain in PHN.

ACTIVITY

- Condom use during sexual activity (in patients with genital herpes)

NUTRITION

- High-lysine diet

Two diseases can arise from VZV: chickenpox and herpes zoster, also called shingles. Chickenpox spreads as an airborne virus. Although not usually a severe illness in childhood, chickenpox poses a greater risk to adults and immunocompromised patients. After chickenpox heals, the virus remains in the body and may reappear years later as herpes zoster. Lesions occur along the distribution of a nerve, usually on the trunk but sometimes on the face or extremities.

POTENTIAL COMPLICATIONS
- Visual impairment and blindness
- Spontaneous abortion
- Hearing loss
- Loss of taste
- Postherpetic neuralgia (PHN)

TREATMENTS

Herpes simplex
- Burow's solution compresses
- Sun block and lip balm when outdoors

Herpes zoster
- Cool compresses
- Zinc oxide lotions (to relieve pain and dry lesions)

RISK FACTORS

Herpes simplex
- Sunlight
- Stress
- Menstrual period
- Trauma
- Systemic infection

Herpes zoster
- Age (adults over age 50)
- Emotional stress
- Immunosuppressive drugs
- Fatigue
- Radiation therapy

AFTERCARE
- Explain to the patient that no treatment can as yet eradicate the virus but that medications can prevent or shorten outbreaks.
- Tell the pregnant patient with genital herpes that the doctor may recommend a cesarean section if she has a positive culture and active lesions at the time of delivery.
- Offer emotional support as needed to the patient with genital herpes.
- Tell the patient to seek help if the following occur:
  – blisters
  – VZV lesions on the face.

IMPETIGO

Impetigo is a purulent and contagious bacterial skin infection. Two types occur: bullous, caused by *Staphylococcus aureus*, and nonbullous, caused by group A beta-hemolytic streptococcus and *S. aureus*. Although the mode of transmission of these bacteria isn't fully understood, direct contact and contamination of clothing play a part. Crowded living conditions and poor hygiene contribute to outbreaks.

Bullous impetigo starts as small, itchy vesicles that appear mostly on the face and trunk. These vesicles — which are filled with fluid that at first appears clear and then turns cloudy but not purulent — enlarge and may remain intact for days. Eventually, the vesicles rupture, leaving behind lesions covered in a thin brown crust.

TEACHING TOPICS

MEDICATIONS

- Topical antibiotics (such as mupirocin) combat infecting bacteria.
- Systemic antibiotics (such as dicloxacillin, cephalexin, and penicillin) combat bacteria.

ACTIVITY

- Regular aerobic exercise (to promote circulation and general well-being)

NUTRITION

- Healthy diet based on recommended portions of the food pyramid

Nonbullous impetigo produces itchy lesions, typically on the legs or arms. The infection starts as small, pus-filled vesicles, which then rupture, leaving a thick, golden crust of dried exudate. Scratching can spread the infection. Treatment for both types of impetigo consists of systemic or topical antibiotics.

POTENTIAL COMPLICATIONS
- Cellulitis
- Septicemia
- Staphylococcal scalded skin syndrome
- Poststreptococcal acute glomerulonephritis
- Scarlet fever

TREATMENTS
- Gentle washing with antibacterial soap and water several times a day; no scrubbing
- Soaks to remove crusts
- Trimming of children's fingernails

RISK FACTORS
- Age (children under age 10)
- Season (higher incidence in summer)
- Location (higher incidence in hot, humid climates)
- Breaks in skin integrity (from insect bites, minor trauma, or other skin disorders)
- Poor hygiene

AFTERCARE
- Tell the patient to disinfect his bedding and towels.
- Tell the sexually active female patient to stop using oral contraceptives (if applicable) and to use another contraceptive while taking antibiotics (antibiotics can prevent oral contraceptives from working).
- Tell the patient to seek help if the following occur:
  – fever
  – blisters or rash on the face or elsewhere on the skin
  – discolored or foul-smelling urine.

PRESSURE ULCERS

Pressure ulcers, also called bedsores or decubitus ulcers, occur commonly in immobilized, malnourished, debilitated, incontinent, and acutely ill patients. Although preventable, these painful, easily infected areas of skin breakdown can form easily and don't heal readily.

As the name implies, pressure ulcers form from excessive pressure on the skin, particularly over bony areas. When compressed between the bone and the external pressure, the skin and underlying tissues break down and become ischemic and necrotic. Other factors that contribute to the formation of pressure ulcers include friction and shearing and moisture. Primary sites include the sacral area and the heels, followed by the buttocks and hips. However, a pressure ulcer can develop on any area subjected to constant pressure or friction.

TEACHING TOPICS

MEDICATIONS

- Vitamin A, B, C, D, E, and K supplements (typically a daily multivitamin) help sustain nutritional status and healing.

ACTIVITY

- Turning at least every 2 hours (more often if needed)
- Use of ergonomic, safe turning techniques
- Active and passive range-of-motion exercises

NUTRITION

- High-calorie or high-protein diet as needed, with nutritional consult
- Vitamins and mineral supplements as needed
- Adequate fluid intake

Pressure ulcers can be classified by the degree of skin breakdown. A stage I ulcer consists of a reddened or purplish area of warm, intact skin that won't blanche. By stage II, the ulcer has broken through the epidermis, possibly to the dermis, and the area may be painful and swollen. A stage III ulcer may extend down to the fascia of the muscle and looks like a deep crater, possibly with overhanging edges; the wound may also have some drainage. By the time an ulcer reaches stage IV, muscle and bone damage and tissue necrosis have occurred, and the wound may drain and have a foul odor.

Pressure relief — the first line of defense — and maintaining good circulation and an adequate diet can keep tissue healthy.

POTENTIAL COMPLICATIONS
- Osteomyelitis
- Sepsis

TREATMENTS
- Achieving and maintaining appropriate weight
- Massaging nonulcerated skin to encourage blood circulation
- Use of dressings, gels, or ointments; may be covered by various occlusive dressings
- No antiseptic solutions
- Use of special mattresses and pads
- Fluidized beds
- Surgical debridement
- Regular, gentle skin and perineal care and thorough, gentle cleaning after bladder or bowel incontinence
- "Moon boots" for heel protection

RISK FACTORS
- Prolonged pressure to the skin (as can occur in bedridden patients)
- Skin shearing
- Moisture
- Immobility
- Incontinence
- Malnutrition

AFTERCARE
- Tell the caregiver to:
  – practice good body mechanics and use turning sheets, a hydraulic lift, and other devices as needed to avoid back strain
  – determine wound depth by gently inserting a cotton-tipped swab and then measuring it with a ruler
  – keep sheets smoothed and free from crumbs and other debris
  – avoid too many layers of padding.
- Tell the patient or caregiver to seek help if the following occur:
  – purulent or bloody drainage
  – fever
  – continued loss of weight by an underweight patient
  – a new sore.

PSORIASIS

A chronic disorder, psoriasis causes noninfectious, inflammatory, papulosqua-mous skin lesions. A patient with this disorder may suffer periodic, possibly disfig-uring flare-ups. Types of psoriasis include psoriasis vulgaris, the most common type; guttate psoriasis, which may follow streptococcal pharyngitis; and pustular psoriasis, which affects the palms and soles.

Although the cause isn't known, it appears to be linked to the immune system. Environmental factors (such as trauma, sunburn, and surgery) can also play a role in triggering an exacerbation, as can certain medications (such as lithium), infections (such as streptococcal infections), and emotional stress. The disorder typically affects the scalp, elbows, knees, buttocks, fingernails, and toenails. Once

TEACHING TOPICS

MEDICATIONS

- Topical steroids decrease in-flammation and itching.
- Psoralens have a photosensi-tizing action on skin cells and are used in conjunction with ultraviolet A.
- Topical and systemic retinoids reduce scaling.
- Topical keratolytics slow skin growth and relieve inflamma-tion, itching, and scaling.
- Antineoplastic agents slow epidermal cell growth and re-duce inflammation.
- Immunosuppressants treat se-vere psoriasis that hasn't re-sponded to other therapies.
- Omega-3 fish oils reduce in-flammation.
- Nonsteroidal anti-inflamma-tory drugs reduce arthritic pain.
- Antihistamines reduce in-flammation and itching.

ACTIVITY

- Minimizing expo-sure to sunlight and using sunblock (es-pecially if taking methotrexate); sun-light may aggravate psoriasis
- Identifying and avoiding triggers
- Regular low-impact aerobic exercise (es-pecially for patients with arthritis)

NUTRITION

- Adequate fluid intake (to maintain skin hy-dration)
- Healthy diet based on recommended por-tions of the food pyra-mid

a flare-up occurs, the patient may have lesions for weeks or months. The epidermal cells in the affected areas grow rapidly and die, resulting in thick, silvery, itchy scales. Removal of a scale reveals a small dot of blood underneath.

No cure exists for psoriasis. Symptomatic treatment consists of some combination of topical or systemic medications and phototherapy, depending on the part of the body affected, the extent and thickness of the plaques, and the patient's response to and ability to tolerate treatment.

POTENTIAL COMPLICATIONS
- Total body erythema and exfoliation
- Arthritis

TREATMENTS
- Achieving and maintaining appropriate weight
- Humidifier use
- Maintaining a cool environment
- Damp dressings and soaks to decrease itching
- Use of fatted soaps and emollients applied to damp skin
- Manual debridement of scales after hydrating
- Ultraviolet phototherapy several times a week; then maintenance
- Psoralens plus ultraviolet A radiation
- No scratching
- Stress management and relaxation techniques, coping skills, music therapy, and massage

RISK FACTORS
- Family history of psoriasis
- Certain medications (antimalarials, beta blockers, iodides, lithium, phenylbutazone, progesterone, salicylates)
- Streptococcal pharyngitis

AFTERCARE
- Tell the patient taking oral methoxsalen to wear special dark glasses for 24 hours to prevent photoactivation of the drug in the eyes, which could lead to keratitis or cataract formation.
- Tell the patient taking methotrexate or cyclosporine that he'll need to have his liver function monitored.
- Tell the female patient taking retinoids to avoid pregnancy.
- Offer emotional support and suggest counseling, as appropriate.
- Tell the patient to seek help if the following occur:
  – drainage from lesions
  – extension of lesions
  – fever.

SCABIES AND LICE

The mite *Sarcoptes scabiei* generally spreads from one person to another by skin-to-skin contact, but mites can also live on furniture and in clothes and bedding for 2 to 3 days.

The host may not notice the infestation for up to a month because the itching and rash that draw the host's attention to the infestation doesn't set in until the body develops an immune response to the mites' saliva and feces. Once the immune response occurs, it kills off many of the mites. However, in a patient with a weak or absent immune response, the mites continue to flourish.

Hallmark signs of scabies include a rash with intense itching that worsens at night and a white line, often with a black speck (the mite) at one end. Skin lesions — usually papules and pustules and, in children, vesicles — typically appear between the fingers, around the wrists, in the armpits, on the areolae of the breasts, and on the buttocks and genitals.

TEACHING TOPICS

MEDICATIONS

- Scabicides and pediculicides, available as lotions, creams, and shampoos, kill both mites and lice.
- Cholinesterase inhibitors (such as physostigmine ophthalmic ointment) can be applied to eyelashes.
- Precipitated sulfur in petroleum can be used to combat infestations in pregnant women or nursing mothers.
- Systemic or topical antibiotics combat secondary infections.
- Antihistamines reduce inflammation and itching.
- Topical steroids reduce inflammation and itching.

ACTIVITY

- Regular aerobic exercise

NUTRITION

- Healthy diet based on recommended portions of the food pyramid

Three types of lice live and multiply on human hosts: *Pediculus humanus capitis*, the head louse; *Pediculus humanus corporis*, the body louse; and *Phthirus pubis*, the pubic or crab louse. Like mites, lice spread by close contact with an infected person but can survive for short periods on bedding and clothing. A person can easily catch head lice by contact with an infected individual or by sharing combs, brushes, or hair decorations such as bows. Pubic lice generally spread by sexual contact, although a person can also catch them by sharing infected sheets or towels. Itching, the presenting symptom, is frequently worse at night. The lice are also big enough to be seen moving around. Other signs include papules, macular and urticarial lesions (in body lice) and, possibly, dry, scaly skin.

POTENTIAL COMPLICATIONS
- Secondary bacterial infection
- Sepsis
- Typhus, relapsing, and trench fever (with body lice)

TREATMENTS
- Applying medicated lotion, cream, or shampoo
- No sharing of combs, hairbrushes, hats, or hair decorations
- Washing clothes and bed linens in hot water

RISK FACTORS
- Weakened or absent immune response
- Chemotherapy

AFTERCARE
- Tell the patient that:
  – preparations of sulfur in petroleum have an unpleasant odor and may stain clothes and sheets
  – itching from scabies will continue for 2 to 4 weeks after treatment.
- Tell the sexually active female patient to stop using oral contraceptives (if applicable) and to use another contraceptive while taking antibiotics (antibiotics can prevent oral contraceptives from working).
- Tell the patient to seek help if the following occur:
  – signs and symptoms of secondary infection
  – signs and symptoms of overtreatment.

VENOUS STASIS ULCERS

Venous stasis ulcers develop when venous congestion secondary to chronic venous insufficiency causes tissue deterioration. Valvular incompetence, thought to be the main cause of the insufficiency, usually develops following deep venous thrombosis. The thrombus slowly reabsorbs, leaving behind damaged valves that can't close properly, thereby causing reflux. This, in turn, allows high venous pressures to reach the tiny venules. The high pressure in the venules, in conjunction with poorly nourished surrounding tissues, results in skin breakdown and venous stasis ulcers.

Venous ulcers usually develop around the ankles, most often on the inner aspect. The skin of the lower extremities of the patient with chronic venous insuffi-

TEACHING TOPICS

MEDICATIONS

- Topical antibiotics (such as neomycin-polymyxin-bacitracin, polymyxin-B, polymyxin-B-trimethoprim, gentamicin, and tobramycin) eradicate bacteria.
- Topical steroids (such as fluocinolone, halcinonide, and triamcinolone) reduce inflammation and itching.
- Systemic antibiotics specific to the infecting organism combat secondary infections.
- Diuretics (such as furosemide) used initially reduce lower extremity swelling.

ACTIVITY

- Possibly bed rest during the acute edematous, weeping phase
- Range-of-motion exercises (even on bed rest) to maintain venous circulation
- No prolonged standing or sitting when the patient becomes ambulatory (to avoid worsening venous stasis)
- Elevating legs when sitting; no crossing legs for long periods
- Regular, gentle aerobic exercise after the acute period (to assist venous return); less exercise if legs swell

NUTRITION

- Healthy diet based on recommended portions of the food pyramid
- Reduced-sodium diet
- Possibly reduced-calorie diet for the overweight patient
- High-fiber diet (to avoid constipation and straining at defecation)

ciency becomes leathery, dry, scaly, itchy, warm, and brown. The patient's lower extremities may swell, and varicose veins and cellulitis with erythema may become obvious. However, he doesn't lose hair on the lower extremities as he would with arterial occlusive disease. Pain or discomfort typically occurs in the lower extremities when the patient stands; elevating the legs above the level of the heart usually relieves the pain.

POTENTIAL COMPLICATIONS
- Septicemia
- Recurrent cellulitis
- Loss of a leg

TREATMENTS
- Achieving and maintaining appropriate weight
- Elastic compression stockings
- Dressing changes (with mechanical debridement)
- Moisture-permeable dressing during the subacute phase, held in place with an elastic compression stocking; no occlusive dressing for a weeping ulcer
- Unna's boot
- Moisturizing creams, ointments, and lotions
- Elevating foot of bed 4″ to 6″ (10 to 15 cm), with doctor's approval
- Smoking cessation
- Surgical debridement
- Skin grafting or venous reconstructive procedures

RISK FACTORS
- Varicose veins
- Deep vein thrombosis
- Venous insufficiency
- Heart failure
- Obesity

AFTERCARE
- Tell the patient to observe safety precautions to avoid further injury to lower extremities.
- Tell the female patient to stop using oral contraceptives (if applicable) and to use another contraceptive while taking antibiotics.
- Tell the patient to seek help if the following occur:
  – purulent drainage from ulcers or from under the Unna's boot
  – swelling of or change in color or temperature of lower extremities
  – new areas of skin breakdown
  – fever.

COPING

Coping is the ongoing process of dealing with stress through mental, emotional, spiritual, and physical efforts. The diagnosis of cancer introduces an enormous stress into the lives of a patient and his family, and the uncertainty and loss of control that cancer brings makes the task of coping that much more complicated.

Cancer requires not only the patient himself to cope but also his family and close friends, and often a wider circle of relatives, coworkers, and members of the patient's religious community. The patient faces the possibility of a changed life, a changed body, disability, disfigurement, and possibly death, along with worries about the costs of treatment. The family must deal with the patient's disability and possible death, role changes, and financial considerations, and learn how to talk about these issues.

TEACHING TOPICS

MEDICATIONS

- Antidepressants (such as amitriptyline, bupropion, trazodone, fluoxetine, paroxetine, sertraline, venlafaxine, and nefazodone) relieve depression.
- Nonnarcotic and narcotic analgesics as needed and prescribed by the doctor can help relieve pain.

ACTIVITY

- Regular aerobic exercise as tolerated
- Active or passive range-of-motion exercises if more strenuous exercise isn't possible
- Alternating activity with rest to prevent overexertion
- Continuing hobbies and interests as possible
- Spending time outdoors when possible
- Adequate sleep

NUTRITION

- Healthy diet based on recommended portions of the food pyramid
- Incorporating favorite foods as appropriate, especially when feeling good

One vital component of coping is whether the patient has the will to live, which can energize him to marshal his forces and fight for the best outcome. A patient without the will to live may cope poorly and exhibit maladaptive behaviors. He may passively accept the situation, refuse to cooperate with or actively interfere with treatment, withdraw, and act in ways that alienate family, friends, colleagues, and health care professionals.

The health care professional can help the patient cope by assessing the patient's needs and providing information and ongoing emotional and spiritual support.

POTENTIAL COMPLICATIONS
- Hopelessness
- Depression
- Loss of the will to live
- Suicidal ideation

TREATMENTS
- Finding meaning in illness
- Developing problem-solving skills
- Developing empowerment and assertiveness skills
- Expecting and accepting the need to grieve
- Education
- Humor
- Spending time alone
- Positive thinking
- Talking over concerns with trusted professionals and friends
- Involvement in interests and hobbies
- Finding comfort and reassurance from support systems
- Interacting with and caring for pets
- Volunteering
- Stress management and relaxation techniques

RISK FACTORS
- Absent or poor support systems
- History of poor coping skills
- Depression
- Pain

AFTERCARE
- Suggest to the patient that a support group can provide emotional support and practical information and that such groups have been shown to increase life expectancy; keep in mind that not all patients benefit from support groups.
- Offer emotional support to the patient and family; suggest counseling as appropriate.
- Tell the patient to seek help if the following occur:
  – thoughts of suicide
  – overwhelming anxiety
  – incapacitating depression
  – pain unrelieved by analgesics.

DIARRHEA

Diarrhea is the frequent passage of loose, watery stool, usually the result of increased peristalsis. The stool may have mucus, blood, or pus in it, and the patient may feel abdominal pain, cramping, and urgency. The main dangers of diarrhea are dehydration and electrolyte imbalances. The cancer patient, who may have chronic diarrhea, may also suffer a loss of appetite from the GI discomfort and the anticipation of diarrhea — making diarrhea one more obstacle in the effort to maintain adequate nourishment.

In the cancer patient, diarrhea can result from several causes: the disease itself; accompanying GI conditions such as pancreatic insufficiency; surgery, such as gastrectomy or intestinal resection; radiation therapy, which can injure cells in

TEACHING TOPICS

MEDICATIONS

- Antidiarrheals (such as bismuth subsalicylate, diphenoxylate, kaolin, and loperamide) inhibit diarrhea.
- Antispasmodics (such as tincture of opium, belladonna, dicyclomine, and hyoscyamine) reduce cramping.

ACTIVITY

- Regular aerobic exercise as tolerated
- Minimizing activity after meals (activity may bring on diarrhea)
- Planning activities so that a bathroom is available

NUTRITION

- Low-fiber diet (may reduce the number of stools)
- Clear liquid diet as needed (to allow GI tract to rest)
- Limited milk and milk products; yogurt is least likely to induce diarrhea
- Increase fluid intake (to prevent dehydration)
- Small, frequent meals (may lessen diarrhea)

the GI tract; and medications, such as chemotherapeutic agents, narcotic analgesics, and antibiotics. Tube feedings can also cause diarrhea.

Treatment includes antidiarrheal and antispasmodic medications, dietary changes, and maintaining hydration.

POTENTIAL COMPLICATIONS
- Dehydration
- Electrolyte imbalance
- Malnutrition

TREATMENTS
- Achieving and maintaining appropriate weight
- Gentle, thorough cleaning of anal area after each stool (helps prevent skin breakdown and infection and keeps the patient more comfortable)
- Applying soothing, protective ointments to anal area after cleaning
- Stress management and relaxation techniques and biofeedback
- Heating pad on low setting placed over abdomen (reduces soreness or discomfort)
- Warm sitz baths (may soothe excoriated or sore anal area)

RISK FACTORS
- Surgery (pyloroplasty, gastrectomy, intestinal resections)
- Radiation therapy
- Chemotherapy
- Antibiotics
- Tube feeding

AFTERCARE
- Tell the patient to:
  – weigh himself daily (at the same time, on the same scale, wearing the same amount of clothing), record weights, and report sudden or steady changes
  – use antacids that contain aluminum; magnesium antacids can worsen diarrhea.
- Tell the patient to seek help if the following occur:
  – weight loss
  – abdominal pain or distention
  – blood or pus in stool
  – fever
  – skin breakdown around anus.

FATIGUE

Cancer patients consistently report that cancer-related fatigue is excessive and out of proportion to energy expenditure. This common and distressing symptom affects the entire body, sometimes interfering with concentration and memory. Rest and sleep don't necessarily relieve the fatigue; in fact, they can make it worse.

Cancer therapies themselves — such as chemotherapy and radiation — provoke fatigue, as do diagnostic tests, nausea and vomiting, and being transported to and from tests and treatments. However, the fatigue described by cancer patients goes beyond that. Several theories try to explain the cause and nature of this tremendous, debilitating, emotionally draining fatigue. One theory ascribes the fatigue to chemical transmission abnormalities, either in the brain or the neuromuscular junctions; another, to metabolic changes at the cellular level, such as lowered glycogen levels in muscle cells; and a third, to bone marrow suppression.

TEACHING TOPICS

MEDICATIONS

- Vitamins (such as a daily multivitamin) to help maintain nutrition.
- Hypnotics (such as temazepam, triazolam, and zolpidem) can relieve insomnia.
- Antidepressants (such as amitriptyline, bupropion, trazodone, fluoxetine, paroxetine, sertraline, venlafaxine, and nefazodone) relieve depression.

ACTIVITY

- Alternating activity with rest to prevent overexertion; stopping activity when symptoms of tiredness occur
- Regular aerobic exercise
- Keeping a fatigue diary
- Planning activities for higher energy times
- Naps as needed
- Adequate sleep at night
- Allowing family and friends to help with tasks and transportation when possible
- Adjusting work schedules as needed
- Energy-conservation measures
- Continuing hobbies and interests as possible
- Spending time outdoors when possible

NUTRITION

- Healthy diet based on recommended portions of the food pyramid
- Nutritional, high-calorie protein supplements as needed
- Small, frequent meals (may be less tiring)
- Adequate hydration

One frequently cited theory suggests that the fatigue stems from the accumulation of wastes from the death of cancer cells in response to treatment.

Whatever the cause, the fatigue is real — and depression, anxiety, stress, pain, nausea, vomiting, and diarrhea compound its effects. The patient's physical condition before the diagnosis also has an impact on how much fatigue the patient experiences.

The patient may take comfort in learning that, in most cases, the fatigue does lift, usually within a year after the completion of treatment.

POTENTIAL COMPLICATIONS
- Loss of self-esteem
- Social isolation
- Depression
- Hopelessness
- Decreased ability to cope

TREATMENTS
- Stress management and relaxation techniques, distraction, and meditation
- Humor
- Music therapy
- Oxygen therapy
- Red blood cell transfusion

RISK FACTORS
- Chronic illnesses (diabetes mellitus, hypertension)
- Pain
- Chemotherapy
- Radiation therapy
- Biotherapy
- Anxiety

AFTERCARE
- Suggest that the patient participate in a support group.
- Tell the patient to seek help if the following occur:
  – worsening fatigue
  – unrefreshing sleep
  – depression that interferes with functioning.

NAUSEA AND VOMITING

Nausea is the distressing gastric queasiness, usually accompanied by increased salivation, that typically precedes vomiting. The vomiting center and chemoreceptor trigger zone in the brain control both nausea and vomiting. In anyone, nausea and vomiting can contribute to loss of appetite, dehydration, and electrolyte imbalances and depletion. In the cancer patient, the nausea and vomiting that recur throughout treatment can significantly hinder the patient's attempts to stay nourished.

Nausea and vomiting in the cancer patient can stem from several different sources. The cancer itself (brain metastases, for example) may cause nausea and vomiting, as can pain medications, such conditions as gastritis and abdominal distention, and such treatments as surgery and radiation therapy. The most common cause, however, is chemotherapy. Some medications (cisplatin, cytarabine, dacarbazine, ifosfamide, mechlorethamine, streptozocin, and cyclophosphamide)

TEACHING TOPICS

MEDICATIONS

- Antiemetics (such as ondansetron, granisetron, prochlorperazine, and metoclopramide) decrease or prevent nausea and vomiting.
- Steroids (such as dexamethasone and methylprednisolone) relieve nausea and increase the effectiveness of antiemetics.
- Cannabinoids (such as marijuana and dronabinol) inhibit nausea and vomiting.
- Antianxiety agents (such as lorazepam) relieve anxiety, helping prevent anticipatory nausea and vomiting before treatment.

ACTIVITY

- As tolerated (patients with significant nausea may have little energy)

NUTRITION

- No spicy or greasy foods (may worsen nausea and vomiting in some patients)
- Eating slowly (may prevent gas or heartburn)
- Possibly eating prepared foods (cooking odors may stimulate nausea and vomiting)

trigger more severe nausea, but many chemotherapeutic agents cause some nausea and vomiting. Many patients experience such unrelenting nausea and vomiting following chemotherapy that they develop anticipatory nausea and vomiting before treatments.

Antiemetics obviously play an important part in managing nausea and vomiting. Understanding and treating both physiologic and psychological factors can help make the patient's nausea and vomiting manageable.

POTENTIAL COMPLICATIONS
- Electrolyte depletion
- Malnutrition
- Dehydration
- Mallory-Weiss syndrome
- Aspiration pneumonia
- Esophageal rupture

TREATMENTS

- Hypnosis, behavior modification, desensitization, guided imagery, biofeedback, relaxation techniques, diversion, music therapy, acupressure, and acupuncture
- Taking antiemetics about 30 minutes before chemotherapy
- Antiemetic suppositories (used after vomiting has begun)

RISK FACTORS

- Certain chemotherapeutic agents (cisplatin, cytarabine, dacarbazine, ifosfamide, mechlorethamine, streptozocin, cyclophosphamide)
- Anxiety
- Anticipatory nausea and vomiting

AFTERCARE

- Tell the patient to seek help if the following occur:
  – weight loss
  – worsening nausea and vomiting
  – dehydration.

NUTRITION

Nutrition supplies the basic energy the body needs to function and maintain weight. It also has other less obvious but vital functions, such as helping the body to maintain its immune response and to recover from injury or illness. In fact, the need for nourishment increases when a person becomes hurt or ill; the body needs energy to heal and to fight off pathogens.

This need for nourishment puts the cancer patient in a catch-22. He needs extra nutrients to contain and destroy malignant cells, but the disease itself, efforts to combat the disease (surgery, chemotherapy, and radiation), pain, and the emotional upheaval that cancer causes can interfere with his ability to maintain even basic nutrition. He may lose his appetite; he may suffer nausea, vomiting, diarrhea, or constipation; foods may taste different; mouth sores or a dry mouth may

TEACHING TOPICS

MEDICATIONS

- Antiemetics (such as ondansetron, granisetron, prochlorperazine, and metoclopramide) prevent or decrease nausea and vomiting.
- Cannabinoids (such as marijuana and dronabinol) inhibit nausea and vomiting and increase appetite.
- Vitamins (such as a daily multivitamin) can supplement nutrition from food.

ACTIVITY

- Activity as tolerated
- Minimizing energy expended on food preparation by using prepared foods or having family members prepare food
- Resting before meals (may help patient eat more)

NUTRITION

- Small, frequent meals
- Increasing calorie intake by adding high-calorie foods
- Adding honey or syrup if foods taste bitter
- High-calorie nutritional supplements
- Making the eating environment as appealing as possible
- Taking pain or antiemetic medications and performing relaxation techniques 30 to 45 minutes before meals
- High-fiber, high-protein, high-potassium, or specialized diet as needed
- Low-fiber diet as appropriate for patients with diarrhea
- Tube, gastrostomy, or parenteral feedings as needed

make eating difficult; his system may not absorb the food well; or he may experience indigestion.

A combination of approaches works best. Medications can help treat pain, mouth sores, malabsorption, nausea and vomiting, diarrhea, and constipation. Coordinating when the patient receives medications with eating and rest periods can optimize nutrition.

POTENTIAL COMPLICATIONS
- Poor healing
- Decreased immunity
- Decreased energy and fatigue
- Malnutrition

TREATMENTS
- Achieving and maintaining appropriate weight
- Tape or dressing changes and skin care for the tube-fed patient
- Dressing changes for the patient on parenteral feedings

RISK FACTORS
- Certain cancers
- Certain chemotherapeutic agents
- Social isolation
- Low income
- Debilitation and loss of mobility

AFTERCARE
- Tell the patient:
  – to weigh himself weekly, record weights, and report sudden or steady changes
  – that he can obtain canned nutritional supplements to take along to drink during long waits or trips away from home.
- Tell the patient to seek help if the following occur:
  – increased appetite loss or decreased food intake
  – fever
  – constipation or diarrhea
  – occurrence or worsening of nausea and vomiting.

PAIN AND DISCOMFORT

Most patients who have cancer experience pain. Many equate the word "cancer" with pain and death. Without careful teaching and reassurance, the fear and effects of pain can overwhelm a patient.

Because it's subjective, pain is hard to describe concretely. Each patient feels it differently, and each patient's life experiences — from culture, to religion, to his emotional and physical state — affect how he perceives and expresses pain.

Depending on the type of cancer, specific treatments, and the patient himself, the patient may experience anything from dull to excruciatingly sharp or piercing pain, and he may have pain from more than one source at any given time.

Methods to help the patient manage pain include assessment tools to gauge his level of pain. Choosing a standardized pain level assessment tool that works best for a particular patient and sticking with that tool throughout treatment can help caregivers and the patient work together to assess his pain accurately. Under-

TEACHING TOPICS

MEDICATIONS

- Analgesics (such as aspirin, acetaminophen, nonsteroidal anti-inflammatory drugs, indomethacin, and ketorolac) relieve mild pain.
- Opioid analgesics (such as morphine, codeine, hydrocodone, oxycodone, hydromorphone, transdermal fentanyl, methadone, and meperidine) relieve or lessen moderate to severe pain.
- Adjuvant analgesics (such as amitriptyline, doxepin, desipramine, nortriptyline, carbamazepine, valproate, gabapentin, clonazepam, baclofen, dexamethasone, dextromethorphan, hydroxyzine, and calcitonin) reduce or relieve specific types of pain.

ACTIVITY

- Range-of-motion and muscle stretching exercises
- Regular aerobic exercise as tolerated
- No hot, loud, or bright conditions (Such conditions may increase pain.)
- Planning necessary or desired activities when pain is under control
- Breathing exercises (to aid relaxation)
- Positioning and frequent turning

NUTRITION

- "Comfort" foods, such as chicken soup, tea and toast, macaroni and cheese, foods brought from home, and warm corn tortillas (Foods will vary for each patient.)

standing how different circumstances and conditions affect the patient's pain can also help the patient manage his pain. For instance, he may simply want a cool washcloth over the eyes, not more pain medication.

No single approach can control a cancer patient's pain. All of the patient's caregivers must work together to understand the patient and respond to his particular needs.

POTENTIAL COMPLICATIONS
- Depression and hopelessness
- Immobility
- Sleeplessness
- Social withdrawal
- Suicidal ideation
- Actual or potential tissue damage

TREATMENTS
- Warm packs or heating pads and ice packs
- Massage, acupressure, acupuncture, transcutaneous electrical nerve stimulation, and biofeedback
- Splints to support painful body parts
- Relaxation techniques, distraction, hypnosis, self-hypnosis, humor, music, prayer, meditation, and imagery
- Keeping a pain-relief record
- Possible administration by patient or caregiver of I.M., I.V., continuous narcotic, or patient-controlled analgesia

RISK FACTORS
- Some cancers (Bone and abdominal cancer cause more pain.)
- Metastases (may invade or compress nerves and invade bones)
- Radiation therapy (may cause skin burns or breakdown and nerve irritation)
- Chemotherapy (may cause peripheral neuropathy, mucositis, and phlebitis)
- Surgery
- Poor coping skills
- Poor support system

AFTERCARE
- Teach the patient how to recognize early signals of pain and start treatment so pain doesn't become overwhelming and incapacitating.
- Explain that opioid analgesics aren't addictive when used correctly for pain management.
- Tell the patient to seek help if the following occur:
  – ineffectiveness of medications
  – intolerable adverse effects of medication.

SKIN AND MOUTH CARE

The largest organ in the body, the skin normally protects the body from infection and provides sensory information. However, in the cancer patient, the integrity of the skin and mouth is at risk.

Cancer results in several threats to the skin. The cancer patient typically has difficulty maintaining adequate nutrition, which leaves the skin vulnerable to breakdown, ulceration, and infection and impairs its ability to heal. The cancer itself may also erode the skin or cause edema. Conditions that may accompany the disease, such as immobility, incontinence, and edema, put the patient at risk for infections and pressure ulcers.

Treatments can also damage the skin and mouth and can result in alopecia, erythema, dryness, flaking, scaling, telangiectasia, thinning, fibrosis, photosensitivity, pigmentation changes, mucositis, infections, and stomatitis.

TEACHING TOPICS

MEDICATIONS

- Systemic and topical antibiotics combat bacterial infections.
- Antivirals combat viral infections.
- Antifungals fight fungal infections.
- Antipruritics relieve or decrease itching.
- Topical steroids relieve inflammation and itching of skin lesions and rashes.
- Anesthetics relieve pain from mouth sores.
- Cannabinoids decrease nausea and vomiting and stimulate appetite.
- Cholinergics stimulate the production of saliva and relieve dry mouth.
- Synthetic saliva and mouth moisteners help relieve dry mouth.

ACTIVITY

- No sunlight on irradiated skin
- No sitting or lying on excoriated, edematous, or broken skin
- Regular aerobic exercise as tolerated (to enhance circulation)
- Active or passive range-of-motion exercises as needed (for immobilized patients)
- Wearing hats and sunglasses when outdoors to protect scalp and eyes (for patients with alopecia)

NUTRITION

- Adequate iron, zinc, and protein (to maintain skin health)
- Adequate fluids (to prevent skin drying)
- Ice chips, ice pops, hard candies, and sugar-free gum (to help relieve dry mouth)
- Soft, nonacidic, moist, smooth, mild foods with no salt; no alcohol (to avoid aggravating mouth sores)

Preventive measures and meticulous care can then help prevent problems or treat problems that arise.

POTENTIAL COMPLICATIONS
- Pain
- Pressure ulcers
- Tissue necrosis and fibrosis
- Infection
- Sepsis
- Decreased ability and desire to eat

TREATMENTS
- Bathing no more than every other day or so with tepid water; can wash or sponge perineal area daily or as needed with mild soap and water
- Mild soap and shampoo
- Cool, humidified environment
- Emollients, oils, creams, and ointments (to soothe dry, itchy skin)
- Premoistened mouth swabs (can soothe and moisturize mouth)
- No mouthwash that contains alcohol, astringents, or phenol
- Soft toothbrush
- Lip balm on lips
- Smoking cessation

RISK FACTORS
- Skin tumors
- Some cancers (Monocytic leukemia; intestinal, colon, and rectal tumors; and salivary gland tumors increase the risk for mucositis and stomatitis.)
- Malnutrition
- Chemotherapeutic agents (Cyclophosphamide, doxorubicin, and vincristine increase risk for alopecia.)
- Radiation therapy
- Immobility
- Decreased immunity

AFTERCARE
- Tell the patient and family to:
  – inspect the patient's skin daily, and look for signs and symptoms of infection or skin breakdown
  – tell the patient's dentist about the diagnosis and treatment; he may need to consult with the oncologist to determine whether the patient's blood counts are acceptable before performing dental procedures.
- Offer emotional support.
- Tell the patient to seek help if the following occur:
  – weight loss
  – skin breakdown or bleeding
  – itching
  – bleeding from gums
  – mouth ulcers
  – fever.

ENDOMETRIOSIS

In endometriosis, endometrial tissue that normally lines the inside of the uterus implants and grows outside of the uterus, usually around the ovaries, fallopian tubes, peritoneum, ureter, bladder, and bowels. This chronic, progressive, and painful disease affects about 10% of women between the ages of 20 and 50.

It's not known why endometrial tissue sometimes grows outside of the uterus. Current theory holds that when endometrial cells reflux through the fallopian tubes during menstruation, they implant and proliferate in the pelvic area. Distant growths — such as in the lungs — may result when a few endometrial cells are transported by the blood or through the lymphatic system. However, it's not known why implantation and growth occurs in some women and not others, especially since some reflux occurs in most women during menstruation. It may result from a combination of the amount of reflux and the effects of steroid hormones and growth factor from the immune and endocrine systems, which stimulate endometrial cell growth.

TEACHING TOPICS

MEDICATIONS

- Nonsteroidal anti-inflammatory drugs (such as flurbiprofen, ibuprofen, and naproxen) decrease inflammation and relieve pain.
- Oral contraceptives suppress ovulation, causing endometriosis to regress.
- Progesterone causes sloughing of the endometrial implants.
- Gonadotropin inhibitors (such as danazol, nafarelin, and leuprolide) suppress ovarian function and cause endometriosis to regress.

ACTIVITY

- Regular aerobic exercise as tolerated (The anemic patient may tire easily.)

NUTRITION

- High-iron diet (to replace iron lost from excessive bleeding)

Once established and growing outside of the uterus, the endometrial tissue responds to the hormonal cycle and bleeds at the end of each cycle. This sets off an inflammatory reaction that eventually leads to scarring, fibrosis, adhesions and, often, decreased fertility or infertility. Because endometrial tissue is hormonally regulated, the disseminated implants don't grow during pregnancy.

Pain, the presenting symptom, starts before menstruation, lasts throughout it, and may continue for another few days. The pain may occur in different parts of the abdomen, depending on the anatomic location of the endometrial implants. The patient may also have heavier, longer, and more frequent menstrual periods than usual as well as pain during defecation and sexual intercourse.

POTENTIAL COMPLICATIONS
- Decrease in or loss of fertility
- Abdominal fibrosis or adhesions
- Peritonitis
- Anemia

TREATMENTS
- Use of a nasal metered pump spray, for patients on nafarelin (Patient should be taught how to use spray.)
- Pain management and relaxation techniques
- Surgical removal of implants
- Bilateral salpingo-oophorectomy (if other methods fail)

RISK FACTORS
- Family history of endometriosis
- Age (women ages 30 to 40, particularly those who have never been pregnant)
- Short menstrual cycles with long menstrual periods
- Delayed childbearing

AFTERCARE
- Tell the patient who wants to get pregnant not to delay pregnancy.
- Tell the patient to seek help if the following occur:
  – increase in amount or frequency of vaginal bleeding
  – abdominal pain or swelling
  – fever.

MENOPAUSE

A normal part of aging in women, menopause — the ending of menstrual cycles — typically occurs between the ages of 45 and 55. Menstruation may stop abruptly, but most women experience a year or two of irregular, variable menstrual periods before menstruation completely stops. A year without any menstrual period signals the start of menopause. For at least the first 6 months of that time, a sexually active woman should use birth control if she doesn't want to get pregnant.

Although a natural process, menopause has certain health consequences. The drop in estrogen levels that normally occurs during menopause coincides with such changes as an increased risk of osteoporosis and heart disease, hot flashes,

TEACHING TOPICS

MEDICATIONS

- Calcium supplements (such as calcium carbonate, calcium gluconate, and calcium citrate) help prevent bone resorption.
- Vitamin D supplements (such as multivitamins, ergocalciferol, and calcifediol) help the body absorb and use calcium.
- Estrogens (such as conjugated estrogen, estropipate, ethinyl estradiol, medroxyprogesterone acetate, and transdermal estradiol) help maintain bone mass.
- Bisphosphonates (such as etidronate and alendronate) slow bone resorption.
- Calcium-regulating hormones (such as calcitonin, given by injection or nasal spray) block bone resorption.

ACTIVITY

- Regular weight-bearing aerobic exercise (slows osteoporosis)

NUTRITION

- High-calcium diet (helps slow osteoporosis)

vaginal atrophy, urinary urgency and frequency, and stress incontinence. Less commonly, uterine prolapse, cystocele, or rectocele may occur.

Estrogen replacement can benefit women during and after menopause, especially by providing protection against cardiovascular disease and osteoporosis. Estrogen replacement can also help ease hot flashes, lessen vaginal atrophy, reduce the effects of urinary problems, and improve skin elasticity and dental health. It may also decrease the risk of Alzheimer's disease.

POTENTIAL COMPLICATIONS
- Osteoporosis
- Higher risk of cardiovascular problems
- Vaginal atrophy

TREATMENTS
- Lubricating creams and topical estrogens for vaginal dryness

RISK FACTORS
Osteoporosis
- Family history of osteoporosis
- Race (higher incidence in Whites and Asians)
- Slender, fine-boned frame
- Early menopause (natural or surgical)
- Cigarette smoking
- High alcohol intake
- Low-calcium, high-caffeine diet
- Sedentary lifestyle

AFTERCARE
- Explain to the patient who has had breast or endometrial cancer, liver disease, or thrombophlebitis that hormone replacement therapy is controversial.
- Tell the patient that she'll need a mammogram before starting estrogen replacement therapy.
- Tell the patient to seek help if the following occur:
  – emotional distress
  – vaginal bleeding after menopause.

PELVIC INFLAMMATORY DISEASE

Pelvic inflammatory disease (PID) — basically a pelvic peritonitis — is an acute inflammation of the uterus, oviducts, ovaries, broad ligaments, bladder, rectum, and pelvic side walls. An infection that ascends upward from the cervix and vagina causes the inflammation, typically a sexually transmitted infection. The microorganisms usually at fault are *Chlamydia trachomatis* and *Neisseria gonorrhoeae*, although streptococci and staphylococci can also cause the disorder.

PID may not cause any symptoms at first and may be discovered during a routine check-up or an assessment of infertility. When signs and symptoms develop, they include lower abdominal and pelvic pain aggravated by defecation, purulent vaginal discharge, abnormal bleeding, pain when urinating, nausea, vomiting, tenesmus, and fever.

TEACHING TOPICS

MEDICATIONS

- Antibiotics (such as cefoxitin, ceftriaxone, doxycycline, and erythromycin) combat infection.
- Narcotic or nonnarcotic analgesics, as prescribed, relieve pain.

ACTIVITY

- No sexual intercourse during treatment
- Bed rest initially as needed, with graduated activity as tolerated

NUTRITION

- Healthy diet based on recommended portions of the food pyramid

Antibiotic therapy is the primary treatment. A patient with a severe infection and pelvic abscesses may need hospitalization and, possibly, surgery. Occasionally, the patient may need to have her uterus, ovaries, and fallopian tubes removed.

POTENTIAL COMPLICATIONS
- Infertility
- Ectopic pregnancy
- Chronic PID
- Peritonitis
- Pelvic abscesses
- Chronic pelvic pain

TREATMENTS
- Warm sitz baths (may be soothing)
- Washing perineum with warm water (to rinse away discharge)
- Wiping perineum front to back after urinating
- Abstinence from sex until treatment is complete
- Surgery if medical treatment fails

RISK FACTORS
- Age (women ages 16 to 25 who have had multiple sex partners)
- Previous episode of PID
- Use of an intrauterine device (IUD)
- Dilatation and curettage or endometrial biopsy

AFTERCARE
- Tell the patient:
  – that any sex partner should receive treatment for infection
  – who has an IUD that she should have it removed
  – not to use douches or vaginal deodorants, which can worsen the infection and remove the normal protective mucosa and flora.
- Tell the patient to seek help if the following occur:
  – worsening of pain
  – fever
  – chills
  – worsening of or a change in vaginal discharge.

POLYCYSTIC OVARY SYNDROME

Polycystic ovary syndrome (PCOS), sometimes called Stein-Leventhal syndrome, is the most common cause of amenorrhea in premenopausal women. The underlying cause of this multifaceted endocrine disorder isn't fully understood, but insulin resistance seems to be a key. Women with PCOS have a higher incidence and greater degree of insulin resistance than other women. This insulin resistance places the women at higher risk for diabetes mellitus and premenopausal cardiovascular disease, including hypertension; it also may be responsible for the hirsutism (from elevated androgen levels) and obesity that can result from PCOS. Other theorists have proposed that PCOS stems from gonadotropin abnormalities. Whatever the specific cause, the result is an imbalance of luteinizing hormone and follicle-stimulating hormone and no ovulation or irregular ovulation and menstrual periods. Eggs, instead of being released from the ovary, fill with immature follicles called cysts and enlarge.

TEACHING TOPICS

MEDICATIONS

- Oral antidiabetics (such as troglitazone and metformin) help reduce blood glucose levels.
- Estrogens (such as conjugated estrogen, estropipate, ethinyl estradiol, medroxyprogesterone acetate, and transdermal estradiol) help maintain bone mass.
- Gonadotropin inhibitors (such as goserelin acetate, leuprolide acetate, and nafarelin acetate) decrease gonadal steroids.
- Androgen inhibitors (such as spironolactone, flutamide, and finasteride) lower androgen levels and reduce hirsutism and acne.
- Antiestrogens (such as clomiphene citrate) encourage pregnancy.

ACTIVITY

- Regular aerobic exercise (for weight loss and general well-being)

NUTRITION

- Reduced-calorie diet (for gradual weight loss)
- Nutritional consult (Insulin resistance makes losing weight difficult.)

The hallmarks of PCOS are irregular menstrual periods, infertility, and hirsutism. Other signs and symptoms include truncal obesity, oily skin, and acne. The patient may have a history of hirsutism and obesity before puberty and of amenorrhea or irregular menses from the time of expected menarche.

Unfortunately, treatment for one set of signs and symptoms may preclude treatment for another. For instance, the patient who wants to become pregnant can't receive treatment for hirsutism because those drugs either suppress ovulation or may damage the fetus.

POTENTIAL COMPLICATIONS
- Infertility
- Ovarian or endometrial cancer
- Insulin resistance and diabetes mellitus
- Hyperlipidemia
- Cardiovascular disease

TREATMENTS
- Achieving and maintaining appropriate weight
- Stress management and relaxation techniques

RISK FACTORS
- Family history of PCOS

AFTERCARE
- Offer the patient emotional support; refer her to counseling and support groups as appropriate.
- Tell the patient to seek help if the following occur:
  – chest pain
  – unusual vaginal bleeding
  – frequent abdominal bloating
  – excessive thirst
  – increased food intake while losing weight.

PREGNANCY-INDUCED HYPERTENSION

About 10% of pregnant women develop pregnancy-induced hypertension (PIH). Gestational hypertension, a relatively benign form of PIH, results in a blood pressure of 140/90 mm Hg or greater after 20 weeks' gestation without edema or proteinuria. A more dangerous form of the disease, preeclampsia includes gestational hypertension but also results in edema and proteinuria. Untreated preeclampsia may escalate to eclampsia, a disorder that threatens the lives of both the mother and fetus.

Although the causes of preeclampsia aren't known, the normal adaptations of the cardiovascular system to pregnancy don't occur. Instead, peripheral resistance

---

TEACHING TOPICS

MEDICATIONS

- Antihypertensives (such as methyldopa, labetalol, and nifedipine) reduce blood pressure, although use of these drugs for mild preeclampsia remains controversial.

ACTIVITY

- Bed rest as indicated

NUTRITION

- Healthy diet based on recommended portions of the food pyramid
- High-protein diet

increases and cardiac output and plasma volume decrease, resulting in decreased perfusion of the placenta, brain, liver, and kidneys.

Preeclampsia ranges from mild to severe. A patient with mild or moderate preeclampsia may be able to remain at home under close monitoring, including fetal nonstress tests in the doctor's office. The patient with severe preeclampsia may need hospitalization and induced delivery.

POTENTIAL COMPLICATIONS
- Heart failure
- Fetal growth restriction
- Placenta abruptio
- Preterm birth
- Fetal death

TREATMENTS
- Maintaining a steady weight gain of not more than 2 lb (0.9 kg) a week
- Daily blood pressure assessment, recording of findings, and reporting of readings outside parameters set by doctor
- Daily urine protein level measurement, reporting levels over 300 mg/dl

RISK FACTORS
- Family history of preeclampsia
- First pregnancy
- Age (higher incidence under age 20 and over age 35)
- Multiple fetuses
- Obesity
- Preexisting hypertension or renal disease
- Diabetes mellitus

AFTERCARE
- Tell the patient to weigh herself daily (at the same time, on the same scale, wearing the same amount of clothing), record weights, and report a gain of more than 2 lb a week
- Tell the patient to seek help if the following occur:
  – contractions
  – rupture of membranes
  – vaginal bleeding
  – nondependent edema
  – severe headache
  – shortness of breath
  – abdominal pain
  – blurred vision
  – vomiting.

PREMENSTRUAL SYNDROME

Premenstrual syndrome (PMS) refers to the group of signs and symptoms that can affect women during the week or two before the onset of menses (the luteal phase). Some women experience only minimal discomfort, but others find that PMS disrupts their daily activities, and a few women become almost incapacitated. Why signs and symptoms and intensity vary so much from one woman to the next isn't understood.

Although the cause of PMS remains unclear, it seems that the monthly fluctuations of estrogen and progesterone influence central nervous system, adrenergic, and serotonin transmitters, resulting in various symptoms that affect several body systems. Mental and emotional symptoms can include irritability and anger, depression, anxiety and tension, withdrawal, crying easily, and mood swings; rarely,

TEACHING TOPICS

MEDICATIONS

- Selective serotonin reuptake inhibitors (such as fluoxetine, sertraline, and paroxetine) taken during the 2 weeks before the onset of menses decreases PMS-related depression, anxiety, irritability, and mood swings.
- Antianxiety agents (such as alprazolam) decrease mental and emotional symptoms.
- Gonadotropin inhibitors (such as goserelin acetate, leuprolide acetate, and nafarelin acetate), administered by subcutaneous injection or nasal spray, decrease gonadal steroids.
- Diuretics (such as spironolactone) help reduce water retention.

ACTIVITY

- Regular aerobic exercise to keep abdominal muscles well toned (helps decrease fluid retention, bloating, and discomfort)
- Keeping a menstrual cycle calendar (foods eaten, activities, dates of physical and emotional changes and menstruation) to determine patterns and factors that trigger signs and symptoms

NUTRITION

- Diet lower in salt, refined carbohydrates, and sugar during luteal phase
- Reduced alcohol and caffeine intake during luteal phase (reduces symptoms in some women)

suicidal thoughts and psychosis occur. Physiologic signs and symptoms typically include water retention, abdominal bloating, constipation, breast tenderness, fatigue, acne, headache, peripheral edema, and food cravings. Flare-ups of migraine headaches and herpes infections may also occur. Many of these signs and symptoms can also result from other disorders, so when they occur during the menstrual cycle can help determine whether they result from PMS.

Treatment usually consists of a combination of medication and dietary modifications during the luteal phase, along with a regular exercise program to tone and strengthen muscles.

POTENTIAL COMPLICATIONS
- Disruption of relationships and regular activities

TREATMENTS
- Achieving and maintaining appropriate weight
- Stress management and relaxation techniques and biofeedback
- Smoking cessation
- Adequate, regular sleep
- Counseling
- Light therapy

RISK FACTORS
- Age (increases with age)

AFTERCARE
- Tell the patient who has had a hysterectomy that she may continue to experience PMS.
- Tell the patient to seek help if the following occur:
  – symptoms interfere with activities of daily living
  – suicidal feelings develop.

VAGINITIS

The most common gynecologic complaint, vaginitis is an inflammation of the vagina. It typically results from bacterial (*Gardnerella vaginalis* and polymicrobial), fungal (*Candida albicans*), or protozoal (*Trichomonas vaginalis*) infections. Other causes include an allergic reaction to a feminine hygiene product or clothing (contact vaginitis) and a lack of estrogen (atrophic vaginitis), typically in postmenopausal women not receiving hormone replacement therapy.

Most patients experience a foul-smelling vaginal discharge, itching, burning, and pain or discomfort during intercourse. Trichomoniasis, which is usually sexually transmitted, produces a greenish-yellow, frothy vaginal discharge. Candidiasis produces a thick, creamy discharge with a yeast-like odor. Bacterial vaginitis re-

TEACHING TOPICS

MEDICATIONS

- Topical steroids decrease inflammation in contact vaginitis.
- Systemic or topical estrogens help control symptoms of atrophic vaginitis.
- Antifungals, available as vaginal creams, ointments, and suppositories, treat candidiasis.
- Systemic or topical antibiotics fight bacterial infections and trichomoniasis.
- Gentian violet paint or tampon combats candidiasis that doesn't respond to topical antifungals.

ACTIVITY

- No sexual intercourse during treatment or, for atrophic vaginitis, the use of condoms if intercourse takes place
- Regular aerobic exercise

NUTRITION

- No alcohol if taking metronidazole (to avoid headache, nausea, and vomiting)
- Healthy diet based on recommended portions of the food pyramid

sults in a thin, watery, grayish discharge with a fishy odor and may not cause much itching or burning. Watery discharge, possibly with flecks of blood, results from atrophic vaginitis; contact vaginitis doesn't usually produce much discharge but does cause itching and burning of the vulva.

POTENTIAL COMPLICATIONS
- Secondary infection from itching

TREATMENTS
- Warm sitz baths (may be soothing)
- Washing perineum with warm water (to rinse away discharge)
- Wiping perineum from front to back after urinating
- Using lubricant during sexual intercourse (in atrophic vaginitis)

RISK FACTORS
- Use of an intrauterine device
- Tight or nylon underwear
- Tight pants
- Antibiotic or long-term steroid treatment
- Diabetes mellitus
- Acquired immunodeficiency syndrome
- Allergic reactions to feminine hygiene products, detergents, soaps, and fabric

AFTERCARE
- Tell the patient:
  – with trichomoniasis that her sexual partners must receive treatment and that she should be reexamined after treatment
  – with bacterial vaginitis that infection during pregnancy may lead to premature rupture of membranes and a low-birth-weight infant
  – to change tampons every 4 to 6 hours
  – not to use douches or vaginal deodorants because they cause irritation and may remove the normal protective mucosa and flora.
- Tell the patient to seek help if the following occur:
  – worsening discharge or itching
  – symptoms that remain or recur after treatment.

ANXIETY DISORDERS

Anxiety is a normal emotional response to a dangerous or stressful situation. Anxiety is considered abnormal when it fails to subside after a stressful situation resolves, its intensity is out of proportion to the triggering event, it interferes with the patient's life and work, and it causes such psychosomatic effects as a dermatitis.

Several types of anxiety disorders can develop. To be diagnosed with *generalized anxiety disorder (GAD)*, the patient must have at least 6 months of chronic, uncontrollable, excessive worry that impairs normal functioning as well as at least three of the following six symptoms: restlessness, fatigue, difficulty concentrating, irritability, muscle tension, and sleep disturbance. *Panic attacks* occur unpredictably and last from 10 to 30 minutes. The patient feels that he may die or go crazy and has feelings of terror and the sense that something awful is about to

TEACHING TOPICS

MEDICATIONS

- Antianxiety agents relieve feelings of stress and worry in patients with panic attacks, GAD, phobias, and PTSD.
- Antidepressants help control panic attacks and GAD when antianxiety medications don't; reduce anxiety in some types of phobias and in OCD; and reduce anxiety and depression in PTSD.
- Beta blockers reduce symptoms of anxiety in social phobia, PTSD, and (occasionally) GAD.

ACTIVITY

- Regular aerobic exercise (helps reduce anxiety and increase feelings of well-being)
- Exercise, walking, or running (can interrupt the progression of anxiety as an attack comes on)
- Adequate sleep

NUTRITION

- Low-tyramine diet for patients taking a monoamine oxidase inhibitor

happen. The attack is accompanied by such physical symptoms as dizziness, chest pain, palpitations, shortness of breath, numbness, and tingling. The fear of negative or embarrassing public experiences can severely limit normal functioning of a patient with a *social phobia*. *Obsessive-compulsive disorder (OCD)* may cause persistent, unwanted thoughts, frequently relating to contamination, illness, violence, religion, or sex. The patient may also feel compelled to perform behaviors that correlate with the obsessive thoughts, including washing, cleaning, counting, checking, or organizing. A patient with *posttraumatic stress disorder (PTSD)* may reexperience an initial traumatic event through nightmares, flashbacks, or intrusive memories and may develop depression.

POTENTIAL COMPLICATIONS
- Panic attacks
- Inability to lead a functional life

TREATMENTS
- Stress management and relaxation techniques
- Deep-breathing exercises
- Thought-stopping techniques (to interrupt phobic or obsessive thoughts)
- Meditation
- Yoga or similar programs

RISK FACTORS
- Gender (higher incidence in women)
- Family history of anxiety (possibly)
- Depression
- Substance abuse

AFTERCARE
- As appropriate, tell the patient:
  – that benzodiazepines may make him feel drowsy for the first few weeks; use caution when driving or doing hazardous jobs
  – that he may not notice the therapeutic effects of buspirone and antidepressants for 2 to 4 weeks
  – not to stop taking an antianxiety agent or antidepressant abruptly; taper off drug according to doctor's instructions to avoid withdrawal symptoms.
- Tell the patient to seek help if the following occur:
  – worsening symptoms of anxiety
  – unmanageable adverse effects
  – behavior dangerous to self or others.

MOOD DISORDERS

The two major types of mood disorders are depression and bipolar disorder, each of which can occur in various forms.

Major depression can occur as a single episode or can recur or become chronic, possibly with psychotic features. Depression can also follow a seasonal pattern (seasonal affective disorder) or occur as postpartum depression. Dysthymic disorder refers to a chronic mild depression without psychotic features. Signs and symptoms of depression include a depressed mood, decreased interest in usual activities, weight loss or gain, changes in sleep patterns, psychomotor agitation, fatigue or loss of energy, feelings of worthlessness or guilt, difficulty concentrating, and thoughts of suicide.

TEACHING TOPICS

MEDICATIONS

- Antidepressants help relieve the symptoms of depression.
- Antimanics, anticonvulsants, and calcium channel blockers stabilize mood in bipolar disorder.
- Stimulants relieve depression from general medical conditions such as acquired immunodeficiency syndrome.

ACTIVITY

- Rising slowly from a sitting or lying position (Antidepressants and calcium channel blockers can cause hypotension.)
- Sunburn precautions if on tricyclic antidepressants
- Regular aerobic exercise (helps relieve symptoms of depression)
- Extra exercise or sports to release excess energy from manic feelings

NUTRITION

- No alcohol if taking an antidepressant (potentiates effects)
- Chewing sugarless gum or sucking hard candy to promote salivation if medication dries mouth
- Low-tyramine or tyramine-free diet if on a monoamine oxidase inhibitor (to prevent hypertensive crisis)
- Increased fluid intake if on lithium
- High-calorie, high-protein diet, with favorite foods to stimulate appetite for manic patient

In bipolar disorders, the patient's mood swings between depression and mania. Cyclothymic disorder is a chronic mood disturbance with periods of hypomania and moderate depression.

Signs and symptoms of mania include an elevated or sometimes irritable mood, inflated self-esteem, decreased need for sleep, talkativeness, racing thoughts or flight of ideas, distractibility, psychomotor agitation, increase in goal-directed activity, and overinvolvement in pleasurable but possibly dangerous activities.

POTENTIAL COMPLICATIONS
- Suicide
- Inability to perform usual functions

TREATMENTS
- Suicide precautions as needed
- Smoking cessation if on tricyclic antidepressants
- Psychotherapy or group, family, or cognitive-behavioral therapy
- Electroconvulsive therapy
- Bright light therapy

RISK FACTORS
- Gender
- Family history
- Anxiety disorders
- Certain medications (for depression, levodopa, amantadine, cimetidine, vincristine, vinblastine, cycloserine, cortisone, estrogen, progesterone; for mania, steroids, amphetamines, tricyclic antidepressants)
- Certain endocrine disorders (adrenal insufficiency, Cushing's syndrome)
- Certain neurologic disorders (for depression, cerebrovascular accident, brain tumor, Parkinson's disease, Huntington's disease)

AFTERCARE
- Tell the patient or caregiver to seek help if the following occur:
  – persistent thoughts of suicide
  – severe headache, nausea and vomiting, seizures, unusual bleeding, chest pain, and priapism (if on trazodone)
  – vomiting, diarrhea, muscular incoordination, blurred vision, tinnitus, tremors, muscle twitching, confusion, or excessive urine output (if on lithium)
  – bleeding, bruising, and skin rashes (if on an anticonvulsant)
  – irregular heartbeat, shortness of breath, dizziness, nausea, and constipation (if on a calcium channel blocker)

PERSONALITY DISORDERS

Personality disorders are individual traits that have become exaggerated and fixed and interfere with daily life. Personality disorders seem to run in families, indicating that some people may have a predisposition to develop such disorders given the right environment and life events. It's thought that a dysfunctional family life can lead to the development of such disorders, laying down characteristics and patterns in childhood that become almost impossible to change.

The American Psychiatric Association (APA) defines three clusters of personality disorders. Cluster A describes odd or eccentric behaviors and includes paranoid, schizoid, and schizotypal disorders. Cluster B behaviors are dramatic, emotional, or erratic and include antisocial, borderline, histrionic, and narcissistic dis-

TEACHING TOPICS

MEDICATIONS

- Antianxiety agents calm agitation in antisocial personality disorder.
- Antipsychotics lessen illusions, obsessive-compulsive symptoms, and phobic anxiety in schizotypal and borderline personality disorders.
- Anticonvulsants and certain antidepressants lessen impulsive, self-destructive behavior in borderline personality disorder.
- Antidepressants also decrease anger and impulsivity and stabilize mood in borderline personality disorder.

ACTIVITY

- Regular aerobic exercise (helps release excess energy and anger)

NUTRITION

- Healthy diet based on recommended portions of the food pyramid
- Low-tyramine or tyramine-free diet if on a monoamine oxidase (MAO) inhibitor to prevent hypertensive crisis

orders. Cluster C refers to anxious or fearful behaviors and includes avoidant, dependent, and obsessive-compulsive disorders; passive-aggressive disorder, once included with cluster C disorders, is no longer listed in the APA class system.

POTENTIAL COMPLICATIONS
- Inability to establish and maintain stable social and occupational relationships
- Self-injury
- Incarceration
- Unstable personal relationships
- Suicide

TREATMENTS
- Learning appropriate means of managing anger

RISK FACTORS
- Family history of the specific type of personality disorder
- Family history of chronic schizophrenia (for paranoid personality disorder)
- Dysfunctional immediate family setting
- Gender (higher incidence of paranoid, schizoid, narcissistic, obsessive-compulsive, and antisocial personality disorders in men; higher incidence of borderline, dependent, and passive-aggressive personality disorders in women)
- Poverty, prepubescent diagnosis of attention deficit hyperactivity disorder, parental deprivation, severe physical abuse during childhood (for antisocial personality disorder)

AFTERCARE
- Tell the patient to seek help if the following occur:
  – behavior dangerous to self or others
  – severe headache, stiff or sore neck, nausea and vomiting, fever, chest pain, palpitations, and dilated pupils (if on an MAO inhibitor).

PSYCHOTIC DISORDERS

Psychotic disorders cause disturbances in perception, thought processes, and behaviors that typically result in social and occupational dysfunction. Patients typically experience episodes of frank psychosis interspersed with variable levels of social and occupational functioning; full recovery rarely occurs.

Initially, the patient (usually in early adulthood) may have some borderline personality attributes that become schizoid in nature, such as emotional limitations, social withdrawal, and aloofness. He then passes through the prodromal phase, exhibiting eccentric behavior, social isolation, lack of initiative, and poor grooming. This phase culminates in schizophrenia with such psychotic signs and symptoms as hallucinations, delusions, and disorganized speech and behavior.

TEACHING TOPICS

MEDICATIONS

- Antipsychotics reduce or relieve psychotic symptoms in both acute and chronic psychoses.

ACTIVITY

- Regular aerobic exercise (to reduce anxiety, increase feelings of well-being, and help prevent constipation)
- Exercise, walking, or running (to interrupt the progression of anxiety as an attack comes on)
- Adequate sleep

NUTRITION

- High-fiber diet (may help prevent constipation, an adverse effect of antipsychotic medication)
- Adequate fluid intake (helps prevent constipation)
- No alcohol while on antipsychotic medication

Types of schizophrenia include disorganized, catatonic, paranoid, undifferentiated, and residual.

Delusional disorder rarely causes hallucinations. Several types exist including *erotomanic, grandiose, jealous, persecutory,* and *somatic* delusion.

POTENTIAL COMPLICATIONS
- Suicide
- Injury to self or others
- Social and occupational dysfunction, with resultant homelessness or incarceration

TREATMENTS
- Occupational rehabilitation
- Social skills training
- Supportive, positive environment
- Stress management
- Smoking cessation as recommended by the doctor (Smoking affects the way antipsychotic medications work.)
- Psychotherapy, behavior therapy, family therapy, social skills training, occupational rehabilitation

RISK FACTORS
- Family history of schizophrenia or other psychotic disorder
- Neurologic disorders (epilepsy, Huntington's disease, parkinsonism, Wilson's disease, cerebrovascular accidents)
- Trauma to the head either during birth or later
- Systemic lupus erythematosus
- Myxedema
- Alcohol abuse
- Personality disorder
- Severe stress

AFTERCARE
- Explain to the patient and his family that:
  – the patient shouldn't stop taking antipsychotic medication abruptly after long-term use; as instructed by his doctor, he should taper off the drug to avoid cardiovascular symptoms
  – the patient should avoid over-the-counter medications without his doctor's approval.
- Tell the patient or caregiver to seek help if the following occur:
  – overtly psychotic symptoms, such as hallucinations or delusions
  – a decline in self-care and coping abilities
  – threatening or dangerous behavior
  – trouble urinating
  – muscle twitching or tremors.

SUBSTANCE ABUSE DISORDERS

The American Psychiatric Association divides substance abuse disorders into two categories: substance-use disorders (abuse and dependence) and substance-induced disorders. These two types of disorders don't have to be interdependent; for example, a patient can experience substance intoxication without being dependent on the substance.

Abuse is defined as the use of a psychoactive drug that has potentially significant health hazards. Dependence (addiction) — whether physical, psychological, or both — is a chronic illness characterized by relapses and overdoses. Intoxication is a reversible, substance-specific syndrome that results from recent ingestion of a substance. Withdrawal, brought on by significantly decreasing or stopping use, results in behavioral, physiologic, and cognitive changes that may render the person incapable of fulfilling social and occupational responsibilities.

TEACHING TOPICS

MEDICATIONS

- Opiate antagonists make the brain's responses to alcohol and cigarette smoking less rewarding.
- Benzodiazepines are used in alcohol and some nonbarbiturate depressant withdrawal.
- Antihypertensives decrease symptoms of opiate withdrawal and help maintain abstinence from alcohol, opiates, and nicotine.
- Antidepressants reduce symptoms in cocaine withdrawal.
- Opiate analgesics reduce withdrawal symptoms and maintain abstinence from heroin.
- Alcohol deterrents produce distressing symptoms, inhibiting impulse drinking.
- Antidepressants and smoking deterrents help patients stop smoking.

ACTIVITY

- Avoiding activities, people, and places associated with substance use
- Renewing or developing other interests and hobbies (to keep the mind and body occupied)
- Regular aerobic exercise (to provide feelings of natural well-being and help maintain general conditioning)

NUTRITION

- Substituting nonalcoholic beverages for alcohol
- Specialized diet as needed (for digestive disorders)
- Healthy diet based on recommended portions of the food pyramid

POTENTIAL COMPLICATIONS
- Industrial and vehicular accidents
- Injuries to self
- Domestic violence
- Sleep disorders
- Brain damage
- Malnutrition
- Cardiac or respiratory arrest
- Infections (such as human immunodeficiency virus) and septicemia
- Depression and psychiatric changes (psychoses, delirium, dementia)
- Fetal damage and dependence

TREATMENTS
- Participation in self-help groups
- Relaxation techniques
- Problem-solving skills
- Counseling and therapy
- Detoxification

RISK FACTORS
- Family history of alcohol abuse
- Abnormal response to drinking alcohol
- Gender (higher incidence of most substance abuse disorders in men)
- Family history of depression (smoking)

AFTERCARE
- Tell the patient, his family, or both that:
  – self-help and support groups can provide support
  – research into vaccines for cocaine use continues.
- Tell the patient trying to quit smoking:
  – not to smoke while using a nicotine patch
  – not to swallow nicotine gum.
- Tell the patient or family to seek help for:
  – nausea and vomiting
  – delirium
  – changes in level of consciousness
  – hallucinations
  – seizures.

PART THREE

APPENDIX, SELECTED REFERENCES, AND INDEX

ACUPUNCTURE

This ancient Chinese method of health maintenance and restoration is based on the theory that channels, or meridians, of energy *(qi)* flow through the body. According to this theory, obstruction of one or more of these 12 meridians results in illness. Inserting and manipulating needles at acupoints — specific places on the body that allow access to the meridians — is thought to unblock and release the flow of energy, restoring the balance of yin and yang and thus restoring health. Because it restores the body's overall balance, treatment for one illness can also result in an improvement in other conditions and in overall health.

In the United States, acupuncture has a growing role as an adjunct to Western medicine. It can reduce or alleviate pain in many conditions, including lower back pain, arthritis, and headaches. Western scientists lean toward the belief that acupuncture relieves pain by either blocking the pain impulses or by stimulating the production of endorphins. Acupuncture can also reduce the desire to smoke in some patients trying to stop smoking and may decrease morning sickness in pregnant women. It can even serve as an anesthetic during surgery for some patients who can't tolerate anesthesia. The needles used vary in size and have rounded rather than pointed tips, allowing them to part rather than pierce tissue. As a result, the patient experiences minimal or no bleeding. Western modifications of acupuncture include electrical stimulation of the needles and laser stimulation of acupuncture points.

Objective

To maintain or restore physical, spiritual, and emotional balance and harmony, thus protecting against illness and helping the body to heal naturally

Instructions for the patient or caregiver

- Make sure you receive treatment only from an experienced acupuncturist.
- Make sure the needles used are sterilized or disposable.

BIOFEEDBACK

Research done in the 1940s has demonstrated that people can use biofeedback to alter physiologic functions once thought to be involuntary, such as heart rate, muscle tension, and blood pressure. This technique uses a mechanical device — such as a beeping monitor or flashing light — to alert the patient to such biologic responses as changes in skin temperature, brainwave activity, sweat gland activity, and preseizure sensations. When the patient learns to recognize these responses, he can learn to modify psychological and physiologic factors to alter them.

Biofeedback can help treat many conditions, including migraine and tension headaches, hypertension, asthma, eczema, chronic pain, premenstrual syndrome, urinary incontinence, cardiac arrhythmias, Raynaud's phenomenon, seizure disorder, and many stress-related conditions.

Objective
To relax, decrease anxiety, and improve health and function by modifying the body's physiologic responses to stress

Instructions for the patient or caregiver
- Check with your doctor to see if biofeedback would be useful for your condition.

CONTINUOUS POSITIVE AIRWAY PRESSURE

A patient with sleep apnea can obtain relief from airway obstruction and maintain upper airway patency during sleep with a continuous positive airway pressure (CPAP) machine, a device that uses a small pump to maintain a flow of air through a mask that fits over the patient's nose. The low pressure of this flow allows the patient to breathe normally but keeps his airways open, eliminating the snoring, choking, and gasping that result from obstruction. Patients who receive CPAP treatment typically experience much more restful sleep, allowing them to stay awake and function more effectively during the day.

Objective
To relieve airway obstruction and allow restful sleep for patients with sleep apnea

Instructions for the patient or caregiver
- To reduce gastric distress, eat a light dinner and then wait at least a couple of hours before going to bed.
- Clip the hose to the pillow or sheet to prevent it from getting tangled during the night.
- Use a heated humidifier or place a small space heater a safe distance from the CPAP air intake to keep the delivered air at a comfortable temperature.
- If you get up during the night, disconnect the hose from the CPAP machine instead of removing the mask (the mask can be hard to reposition).
- If you have trouble adjusting to the mask or develop irritated skin or headaches, make sure the mask is the right size for you. If you still have trouble, try wearing

the disconnected mask on and off during the day to get used to the feel, or use hypnosis to adjust to sleeping in the mask.
- If needed, use a mouth guard to prevent teeth grinding.
- Keep some small mints at the bedside to relieve a dry mouth.
- Take all medications and use nasal sprays as prescribed.

ENERGY CONSERVATION TECHNIQUES

Using techniques to conserve energy can allow the patient with a disorder that drains energy — such as chronic obstructive pulmonary disease — to function as effectively as possible.

Objective
To use techniques that require less energy to manage activities of daily living, thus reducing fatigue

Instructions for the patient or caregiver
- Sit instead of standing when bathing (using a shower or tub chair), washing your face, brushing your teeth, dressing, and working in the kitchen.
- Dry yourself after bathing by wrapping up in a large towel or bath sheet and resting until dry.
- Wear loosely fitting clothes that you can put on and take off easily; choose clothes that use Velcro and elastic rather than buttons and zippers.
- Choose clothes that fasten in the front and are made of nonwrinkling material.
- Choose shoes that don't need to be tied or buckled.
- Use aids to help you dress (such as a sock puller) and fix meals (such as a reacher) to minimize bending over and reaching.
- Keep commonly used items in easy reach, and keep items near where you'll use them.
- Use plastic or paper plates, cups, and utensils; they weigh less and don't need washing.
- Use large and small appliances to do as much meal preparation and housework as possible.
- Don't dry dishes, pots, or pans; let them air-dry.
- Stock up on easily prepared and frozen foods that you can use on low-energy days.
- Use good body mechanics; they're less tiring and help prevent strain and injury.
- Space tiring activities through the day and week, allowing for rest periods and light days in between.

- Allow others or (if possible) hire others to do large, tiring chores, such as heavy cleaning and yard work.
- Take pain medications and breathing treatments shortly before important activities.
- When possible, plan important activities at times when you have the most energy.

HOME SAFETY

Arranging the home to make it as safe as possible for the patient with poor eyesight, osteoporosis, vertigo, or difficulty walking decreases the risk of injury.

Objective
To help prevent injuries from bumps and falls

Instructions for the patient or caregiver
- Maintain good lighting to increase visibility; obtain extra lamps as needed, and promptly replace burned-out bulbs.
- Keep a lamp or working flashlight by the bedside.
- Keep a telephone programmed with emergency numbers by the bedside.
- Remove all throw rugs and rugs without rubber backing; straighten or tack down loose or wrinkled carpet.
- Rearrange furniture as needed to provide a clear pathway.
- Remove any electrical, telephone, or other cords that stretch across the floor.
- Remove any low items that may be hard to see when walking, such as footstools and flowerpots.
- Install safety bars near toilets and tubs.
- As needed, install a raised toilet seat.
- Don't lock bedroom or bathroom doors.
- If necessary, have someone attend the patient in the bathroom.
- Use a shower or tub chair.
- As necessary, use an electric razor instead of a manual one.
- Secure stairway railings.
- As needed, apply nonskid treads at the edges of steps.
- Make sure armchairs are high enough for safe sitting and rising.
- Lock the wheelchair before sitting or rising.
- Use proper body mechanics when lifting, turning, lowering, and positioning (both patient and caregiver).
- As appropriate, keep the side rails up on the bed.

- Set the water heater at or below 110° F (43.3° C).
- Use a heating pad only on the lowest setting.
- Don't smoke unattended or in bed.
- Keep a fire extinguisher readily available and know how to use it.
- Place smoke and carbon dioxide detectors just outside the bedroom.

OXYGEN THERAPY

A liquid oxygen unit, tank, or concentrator allows the patient to receive oxygen at home. The patient usually receives the oxygen through a nasal cannula or mask.

Objective
To improve blood oxygenation, increasing the patient's energy and stamina for activities of daily living

Instructions for the patient or caregiver
- As instructed, set a low flow rate for the patient with chronic lung disease to prevent carbon dioxide narcosis.
- Never set the flow rate higher than prescribed.
- Check the water level on the humidifier about every 8 hours, and fill as needed with sterile water.
- Use a water-soluble lubricant to keep the nasal mucosa from becoming dry and irritated.
- If the oxygen tubing irritates the skin, place a folded 4" × 4" gauze pad between the tubing and the skin at the sides of the head above the ears.
- Make sure that no one smokes and that there are no gas heaters in the room when the patient is receiving oxygen.
- Check all electrical equipment in the room where the patient receives oxygen for frayed cords and sealed connections.
- Keep a fire extinguisher readily available and know how to use it.
- Keep the telephone number of the oxygen supply company by the telephone.
- Tell the fire department that you have oxygen at the home; they may perform a fire safety check.
- Alert the oxygen supply company, airlines, and hotels about the need for oxygen during travel and at the destination; if necessary, the patient can use small canisters for short-term use.
- Plan for a steady supply of replacement oxygen and supplies so the patient is never without oxygen.

RELAXATION TECHNIQUES

The relaxation response causes both physiologic and psychological changes. It can decrease not only oxygen consumption, muscle tone, and heart and respiratory rate but also feelings of anxiety and pain perception.

Several techniques can induce relaxation. Many of them involve finding a quiet environment and comfortable position, adopting a passive attitude, and mentally focusing on a mantra — a single word, sound, or phrase, such as "om" or "peace," that the patient finds calming. Specific relaxation techniques include progressive muscle relaxation, breathing exercises, prayer, meditation, massage, hypnosis, distraction, imagery, aromatherapy, music therapy, yoga, t'ai chi, and (as discussed above) biofeedback. The relaxation response improves with practice.

Objective
To promote healing and decrease stress, anxiety, tension, and pain by relaxing both the body and mind

Instructions for the patient or caregiver
- Talk with your doctor about what relaxation techniques may work best for you.
- Consider any physical limitations when choosing relaxation techniques.

SMOKING CESSATION

Many medical conditions require that a patient who smokes give up smoking. Several smoking cessation methods exist, and the patient may choose a single approach or use some combination of methods.

Nicotine replacement addresses the addiction to nicotine and permits tapering the dosage while avoiding the harmful tar and carbon monoxide contained in tobacco smoke. Nicotine gum is available over-the-counter. Four main brands of the nicotine patch, available in graduated dosages, allow a gradual withdrawal from nicotine. The nicotine inhaler most closely mimics smoking, providing oral gratification with the mouthpiece and hand-to-mouth movements similar to cigarette use. It delivers vaporized nicotine (about one-third of the amount found in cigarettes), which the membranes of the mouth and throat absorb; treatment lasts from 3 to 6 months. Nicotine nasal spray is absorbed through the nasal mucosa and delivers about as much nicotine as a filtered, low-tar cigarette per squirt. It's usually used with decreasing frequency over a 3-month period.

Hypnosis can decrease the patient's desire to smoke as well as cravings associated with nicotine withdrawal. The antidepressant bupropion hydrochloride (Zyban) seems to decrease the craving for nicotine. A motivated patient may be able to quit abruptly and not resume smoking.

Objective

To overcome nicotine addiction and free the patient from nicotine's dangerous effects (cardiovascular in particular) and to keep the patient's lungs free from irritants and carcinogens

Instructions for the patient or caregiver

- Don't use a nicotine replacement method if you're pregnant or breast-feeding.
- If you're using nicotine chewing gum:
  - remember that nicotine is absorbed through the membranes of the mouth, so chew slowly and place the gum between your cheek and gums if it causes tingling or starts to taste peppery
  - don't quickly chew and then swallow the gum or you may develop nausea
  - spit out the gum after about 30 minutes (it will have lost its effect by then)
  - don't chew more than 24 pieces a day.
- If you're using a nicotine patch:
  - don't smoke while wearing the patch
  - don't place a patch on irritated or broken skin
  - change the site daily
  - remove the patch before bedtime (if you're using the 16-hour instead of the 24-hour patch) to help prevent the unpleasant dreams that may occur with the patch in place.

STRESS MANAGEMENT

Stress occurs whenever a person must adapt to the inevitable changes and occurrences of life and produces the normal reaction of anxiety. Each person develops his own unique set of coping mechanisms to deal with stresses and reduce anxiety. Many of these coping mechanisms work well to reduce anxiety but some don't work well or may actually be counterproductive.

Illness and the changes it inflicts on a patient's life produce stress and anxiety that may strain the patient's coping abilities. The level of anxiety the patient feels rests more on his perception of his illness and its repercussions rather than the severity of the illness itself. To help the patient cope with the illness and his reaction to it, the nurse can suggest or help the patient use techniques that may reduce anxiety in positive and productive ways.

Objective

To decrease the negative effects of stress and anxiety and improve the patient's quality of life and ability to function

Instructions for the patient or caregiver

- Learn how to recognize signs and symptoms of stress — increased heart rate, muscle tension, gastric uneasiness, forgetfulness, irritability — and cope with stress in positive ways.
- Maintain a healthy diet that provides adequate nutrients (vitamin supplements may be helpful), and limit intake of caffeine, sugar, junk foods, and preservatives.
- Try to get adequate sleep and rest to help you feel refreshed, renewed, and able to function.
- Spend time communing with nature; suggested activities include gardening, walking by the sea or through the woods or fields, and bird watching.
- If you own a pet, play with, stroke, and interact with it; studies show that such activities lower blood pressure and decrease anxiety.
- Prioritize commitments and responsibilities to help you spend your energy appropriately.
- Use positive thinking to help you accomplish high-priority tasks.
- Take part in physical activities, such as walking, swimming, and housecleaning, to decrease tension and reduce fatigue and anxiety.
- Use relaxation techniques to reverse the physical and mental effects of stress.
- Incorporate laughter and humor in your life by visiting friends, watching appropriate movies and videos, listening to tapes, seeing shows, and so on.
- Try biofeedback to change counterproductive physiologic reactions, such as high blood pressure or muscle tension.
- Participate in a healing, calming, and strengthening system, such as yoga or t'ai chi, to improve mental and physical health.

TRANSCUTANEOUS ELECTRICAL NERVE STIMULATION

A transcutaneous electrical nerve stimulation (TENS) unit delivers a low-voltage electric current through two electrodes placed on the skin. This current is thought to reduce pain either by blocking pain impulses before they travel to the brain or by increasing the body's production of endorphins. TENS can help relieve both acute and chronic pain and seems to work well in relieving postoperative pain.

Objective
To relieve pain

Instructions for the patient or caregiver
- Place the electrodes of the TENS unit over trigger points — particularly sensitive areas, acupuncture points, or spinal nerve roots. You can try the electrodes in different places to see what feels best.
- If needed, dampen the electrodes with water or cover them with a conductive gel before placing them on the skin.
- Don't place electrodes on broken skin or on an area that has a rash.
- Don't use TENS while sleeping; you can use it just before bedtime to decrease pain and promote comfortable sleep.
- Set the controls to regulate the intensity, pulse width, and timing of the electrical pulses.
- Keep the TENS unit dry. If it gets wet, turn it off, disconnect it, and let it dry completely before using it again.
- If the electrical impulses grow weaker, check to see if the unit needs new batteries.
- Gently and thoroughly clean and lubricate the skin after removing the electrodes.

Apple, M.S. *Principles & Practice of Interventional Cardiology.* Philadelphia: Lippincott Williams & Wilkins, 1998.

Arffa, R.C. *Grayson's Diseases of the Cornea,* 4th ed. St. Louis: Mosby–Year Book, Inc.,1997.

Ashton, D., and Richards, A. *Coronary Disease in Women: Aetiology, Diagnosis, Management and Prevention.* Philadelphia: W.B. Saunders Co., 1998.

Beare, P.G. *Adult Health Nursing,* 3rd ed. St. Louis: Mosby–Year Book, Inc., 1998.

Bork, K., et al. *Diseases of the Oral Mucosa and the Lips.* Philadelphia: W.B. Saunders Co., 1996.

Crandell, A.S., and Masket, S. *Atlas of Cataract Surgery.* St. Louis: Mosby–Year Book, Inc., 1998.

Dambro, M.R. *Griffith's 5 Minute Clinical Consult.* Philadelphia: Lippincott Williams & Wilkins, 1999.

Fauci, A.S., et al., eds. *Harrison's Principles of Internal Medicine,* 14th ed. New York: McGraw-Hill Book Co., 1998.

Fonseca, R.J., and Walker, R.V. *Oral and Maxillofacial Trauma,* 2nd ed. Philadelphia: W.B. Saunders Co., 1997.

Gorrrie, T.M., et al. *Foundations of Maternal-Newborn Nursing,* 2nd ed. Philadelphia: W.B. Saunders Co., 1998.

Graham-Brown, R. *Dermatology.* St. Louis: Mosby–Year Book, Inc., 1998.

Ignatavicius, D., et al. *Medical-Surgical Nursing: A Nursing Process Approach,* 2nd ed. Philadelphia: W.B. Saunders Co., 1998.

Kaban, L.B., et al. *Complications in Oral and Maxillofacial Surgery.* Philadelphia: W.B. Saunders Co., 1997.

McKenry, L.M. *Patient Teaching Guides in Pharmacology.* St. Louis: Mosby–Year Book, Inc., 1998.

Middelton, E., et al. *Allergy: Principles and Practice,* 5th ed. St. Louis: Mosby–Year Book, Inc., 1998.

Monahan, F. D., and Neighbors, M. *Medical-Surgical Nursing: Foundations for Clinical Practice,* 2nd ed. Philadelphia: W.B. Saunders Co., 1998.

Palay, D.A., and Krachmer, J.H. *Ophthalmology for the Primary Care Practitioner.* St. Louis: Mosby–Year Book, Inc.,1998.

Patient Education. *HealthCare Professional Guides.* Springhouse, Pa.: Springhouse Corp., 1998.

Pillitteri, A. *Maternal & Child Nursing: Care of the Childbearing and Childrearing Family,* 3rd ed. Philadelphia: Lippincott Williams & Wilkins, 1999.

Professional Guide to Diseases, 6th ed. Springhouse, Pa.: Springhouse Corp., 1998.

Professional Guide to Signs & Symptoms, 2nd ed. Springhouse, Pa.: Springhouse Corp., 1997.

Rakel, R. ed. *Conn's Current Therapy.* Philadelphia: W.B. Saunders Co., 1998.

Redman, B.K. *The Practice of Patient Education,* 8th ed. St. Louis: Mosby–Year Book, Inc.,1997.

Tardy, M.E. *Rhinoplasty: The Art and the Science.* Philadelphia: W.B. Saunders Co., 1997.

Usatine, R., and Moy, R.L. *Skin Surgery: A Practical Guide.* St. Louis: Mosby–Year Book, Inc., 1998.

Weinberger, S.E. *Principles of Pulmonary Medicine,* 3rd ed. Philadelphia: W.B. Saunders Co., 1998.

Wu, G. *Ophthalmology for Primary Care.* Philadelphia: W.B. Saunders Co., 1997.

Zadnik, K. *The Ocular Examination: Measurements and Findings.* Philadelphia: W.B. Saunders Co., 1997.

A

E

Eclampsia. *See* Pregnancy-induced hypertension.

Education, patient. *See also* Assessment, educational needs and; Learning objectives.
 documentation of, 27-28
 evaluation of, 26-27
 process of, 12-28
 reasons for, 2-11
 responsibility for, 2-3, 3t
Enalapril, 170
Endocarditis, 42-43
Endocrine and metabolic disorders, 134-149
Endometriosis, 230-231
Energy conservation techniques, 258-259
English, inability to speak, 24-25, 25t
Ephedrine, 104
Epilepsy. *See* Seizure disorder.
Epinephrine, 186
Epinephrine, anaphylaxis and, 78
Epistaxis, 184-185
Epoetin alfa, 178
Erythromycin, 60, 68, 190, 198, 200, 234
Erythropoietin, 178
Estrogen, 142, 162, 180, 232, 236, 242, 247
Estropipate, 142, 232, 236
Ethambutol, 76
Ethinyl estradiol, 142, 232, 236
Ethosuximide, 108
Etidronate, 232
Etodolac, 160
Expectorants, 62, 66
Eye, ear, nose, and throat disorders, 184-197
Eyedrops, 72

F

Famciclovir, 96, 204
Famotidine, 130
Fatigue, cancer and, 220-221
Felbamate, 108
Fexofenadine, 200
Fibrinolysis inhibitors, 80
Fibromyalgia, 152-153
Finasteride, 168, 236
Flavoxate, 174, 182
Flu. *See* Influenza.
Flucytosine, 68
Fludrocortisone, 134
Flunisolide, 58, 192
Fluocinolone, 214
Fluoxetine, 92, 94, 216, 220, 240

Flurbiprofen, 230
Flutamide, 236
Fluticasone, 192
Fluvastatin, 142
Folic acid, 86, 108
Fractures, 154-155
Fresh frozen plasma, 80
Furosemide, 170, 176, 214

G

Gabapentin, 108, 110, 226
GABHS. *See* Pharyngitis.
GAD. *See* Anxiety disorders.
Gallbladder. *See* Cholecystitis.
Gallstone solubilizers, 112
Gamma interferon, 198
Gastric acid inhibitors, 188
Gastrointestinal reflux disease, 120-121
Gastrointestinal stimulants, 120, 126, 188
Gemfibrozil, 142
Generalized anxiety disorder. *See* Anxiety disorders.
Gentamicin, 118, 214
Gentian violet paint, 242
GERD. *See* Gastrointestinal reflux disease.
Gestational hypertension. *See* Pregnancy-induced hypertension.
Glaucoma, 186-187
Glipizide, 138
Glomerulonephritis, 170-171
Glutamate antagonists, 94
Glyburide, 138
Glycopyrrolate, 112
Gold salts, 91
Gonadotropin inhibitors, 230, 236, 240
Goserelin acetate, 236, 240
Gout, 140-141
Granisetron, 222, 224
Grave's disease. *See* Hyperthyroidism.
Group A beta-hemolytic streptococci. *See* Pharyngitis.

H

Halcinonide, 214
Haloperidol, 92
Hashimoto's disease, 146
HDL. *See* High-density lipoprotein.
Headaches, 100-101
Heart attack. *See* Myocardial infarction.
Heartburn. *See* Gastrointestinal reflux disease.
Heart failure, 44-45

Helping relationship, patient education and, 5
Hemoglobin A, 86
Hemoglobin S, 86
Hemophilia, 80-81
Hemorrheologics, 52, 98
Hemorrhoids, 122-123
Heparin, 38-39, 70
Hepatitis, viral, 124-125
Hepatitis vaccines, 124
Herniated disk, 156-157
Herniated nucleus pulposus. *See* Herniated
    disk.
Herpes simplex and herpes zoster, 204-205
Hiatal hernia, 126-127
High-density lipoprotein, 142-143
Hismanal, itraconazole and, 203
Histamine$_2$-receptor antagonists, 120, 124,
    126, 130, 132
HIV. *See* Human immunodeficiency virus
    infection.
Home care techniques, 256-264
Home safety, 259-260
Human immunodeficiency virus infection,
    82-83
Hydrochlorothiazide, 170, 194
Hydrocodone, 60, 150, 154, 226
Hydrocortisone, 122, 134, 198, 200
Hydromorphone, 156, 174, 226
Hydroxyzine, 198, 200, 226
Hyoscyamine, 218
Hypercortisolism. *See* Cushing's syndrome.
Hyperlipidemia, 142-143
Hypertension, 46-47. *See also* Pregnancy-
    induced hypertension.
Hyperthyroidism, 144-145
Hypnotics, 220
Hypothyroidism, 146-147

IJ

Ibuprofen, 81,156, 164, 166, 230
Ifosfamide, 222-223
Illiterate patient, teaching the, 22-24, 23t
Immune and hematologic disorders, 78-91
Immune globulin, 124
Immune serums, 124
Immunoglobulin G antibodies, 84-85
Immunoregulators, 102, 124
Immunosuppressants, 88, 90, 102, 104, 128,
    170, 210
Impetigo, 206-207
Indomethacin, 50, 140, 166, 226

Inflammatory bowel disease, 128-129
Influenza, 66-67
Insulins, 130, 138
Interferon, 124
Iodines, 144
Ipratropium, 58
Iron supplements, 64
Ischemia. *See* Cerebrovascular accident.
Ischemic heart disease. *See* Coronary artery
    disease.
Isoniazid, 76
Isoproterenol, 58
Isosorbide, 30
Itraconazole, drug interactions with, 203

K

Kaolin, 218
Keratolytics, 198, 210
Ketoconazole, 134, 136
Ketoprofen, 166
Ketorolac, 226

L

Labetalol, 30, 238
Lactulose, 116
Laënnec's cirrhosis. *See* Cirrhosis.
Lamivudine, 82
Lamotrigine, 108
Lansoprazole, 132
Laryngitis, 188-189
Latanoprost, 186
Laxatives, 176
LDL. *See* Low-density lipoprotein.
Learning objectives, 15-16, 16t
Learning styles, types of, 18-19
Leuprolide, 230, 236, 240
Levodopa, 106-107, 247
Levothyroxine, 74, 142
Lice, scabies and, 212-213
Lidocaine, 190, 204
Liothyronine, 142
Lipoprotein, low-density, 142-143
Loop diuretics, 40, 44, 46
Loperamide, 104, 218
Loracarbef, 192
Loratadine, 200
Lorazepam, 92, 222
Lou Gehrig's disease. *See* Amyotrophic lateral
    sclerosis.
Lovastatin, 142, 170
Low-density lipoprotein, 142-143

P

Pain and discomfort, cancer and, 226-227
Pancreatic enzyme supplements, 64
Pancreatin, 130
Pancreatitis, chronic, 130-131
Pancrelipase, 130
Panic attacks. *See* Anxiety disorders.
Parkinson's disease, 106-107
Paroxetine, 92, 216, 220, 240
PCOS. *See* Polycystic ovary syndrome.
Pelvic inflammatory disease, 234-235
Penicillin, 42, 50, 86, 170, 190, 200, 206
Pentamidine, 68
Pentazocine, 150, 154
Pentoxifylline, 52
Peptic ulcer disease, 132-133
Pergolide, 106
Pericarditis, 50-51
Peripheral arterial occlusive disease, 52-53
Periurethral collagen, 180
Personality disorders, 248-249
Pharyngitis, 190-191
Phenazopyridine, 174, 182
Phenobarbital, 108, 134
Phenolphthalein, 116
Phentermine, 142
Phenylephrine, 192
Phenylpropanolamine, 142
Phenytoin, 108, 110, 134, 194
Physostigmine ophthalmic ointment, 212
PID. *See* Pelvic inflammatory disease.
PIH. *See* Pregnancy-induced hypertension.
Pilocarpine, 186
Pituitary hormones, 80
Platelet aggregation inhibitors, 98
PMS. *See* Premenstrual syndrome.
Pneumonia, 68-69
Polycystic ovary syndrome, 236-237
Polymyxin-B, 214
Polymyxin-B-trimethoprim, 214
Postnecrotic cirrhosis. *See* Cirrhosis.
Posttraumatic stress disorder. *See* Anxiety disorders.
Potassium, 116, 122
Potassium-sparing diuretics, 40, 44, 46
Potassium supplements, 40, 44, 46, 56
Pravastatin, 142, 170
Prazosin, 54
Precipitated sulfur in petroleum, 212
Prednisolone, 90, 166

Prednisone, 50, 58, 60, 90, 96, 104, 134, 136, 140, 158, 170, 190, 198, 200, 204
Preeclampsia. *See* Pregnancy-induced hypertension.
Pregnancy-induced hypertension, 238-239
Premenstrual syndrome, 240-241
Pressure ulcers, 208-209
Primidone, 108, 194
Prinzmetal's angina, 31
Probenecid, 140
Procainamide, 72, 91
Prochlorperazine, 196, 222, 224
Progesterone, 230, 247
Promethazine, 196
Propantheline, 174, 182
Propoxyphene, 150, 154, 156, 160
Propranolol, 32, 72
Propulsid, itraconazole and, 203
Prostaglandins, 186
Proton pump inhibitors, 120, 126, 132
Protriptyline, 106
Pseudoephedrine, 192
Psoralens, 210
Psoriasis, 210-211
Psychiatric disorders, 244-253
Psychotic disorders, 250-251
Psyllium, 106, 116, 118, 122
PTSD. *See* Anxiety disorders.
Pulmonary embolism, 70-71
Pyelonephritis, 172-173. *See also* Urinary tract infection.
Pyrazinamide, 76
Pyridostigmine bromide, 104

Q

Quinidine, 72, 91
Quinine, 91

R

Radioiodines, 144
Ranitidine, 120, 126, 130, 132
Raynaud's phenomenon, 54-55
Relaxation techniques, 261
Renal and urological disorders, 168-183
Renal calculi, 174-175
Renal failure
  acute, 176-177
  chronic, 178-179
Respiratory disorders, 58-77
Retinoids, 210

Reye's syndrome, aspirin and, 191
Rheumatoid arthritis, 84-85
RICE protocol, 164-165
Rifampin, 76, 77, 134
Riluzole, 94
Risperidone, 92
Ritonavir, 82
Ruptured disk. *See* Herniated disk.

S

Salicylates, contraindications to, 71, 81
Salsalate, 160
Saquinavir, 82
Sarcoidosis, 72-73
Scabicides, 212
Scabies and lice, 212-213
Schizophrenia. *See* Psychotic disorders.
Seasonal affective disorder. *See* Mood disorders.
Sedatives, 196
Seizure disorder, 108-109
Selective serotonin reuptake inhibitors, 240
Selegiline, 106
Senility. *See* Alzheimer's disease.
Senna, 116
Serotonin selective agonists, 100
Sertraline, 92, 216, 220, 240
Shingles. *See* Herpes simplex and herpes zoster.
Sibutramine, 148
Sickle cell syndrome, 86-87
Simvastatin, 142
Sinusitis, 192-193
Skeletal muscle relaxants, 94, 102, 110, 150, 152, 156
Skin care, cancer and, 228-229
Skin disorders, 198-215
Sleep apnea syndrome, 74-75
Sleeping aids, 92
Slipped disk. *See* Herniated disk.
Smoking cessation, 261-262
Smoking deterrents, 252
Social phobia. *See* Anxiety disorders.
Sodium, 116, 122
Sodium edetate, 72
Somatostatin, 136
Sorbitol, 116, 176
Spironolactone, 112, 136, 236, 240
Sprains and strains, 164-165
Stavudine, 82

Stein-Leventhal syndrome. *See* Polycystic ovary syndrome.
Steroids, 50, 58, 60, 62, 64, 72, 88, 90, 96, 100, 102, 104, 128, 134, 136, 140, 144, 158, 166, 170, 188, 190, 198, 200, 204, 210, 212, 214, 222, 228, 242, 247
Stimulant laxatives, 116
Stimulants, 246
Strains, sprains and, 164-165
Streptokinase, 70
Streptomycin, 42, 50, 76
Streptozocin, nausea, cancer and, 222-223
Stress management, 262-263
Stroke. *See* Cerebrovascular accident.
Struvite calculi. *See* Renal calculi.
Subacute bacterial endocarditis. *See* Endocarditis.
Substance abuse disorders, 252-253
Sulfa, 91
Sulfa derivatives, 91
Sulfamethoxazole, 182
Sulfisoxazole, 182
Sulindac, 160
Sunscreens, 88
Surfactant laxatives, 102, 122
Sympathomimetic drugs, 186, 188
Synthetic saliva, 228
Systemic biological response modulators, 198
Systemic lupus erythematosus, 88-89

T

Tachycardia, 34-35
Tacrine, 92
TB. *See* Tuberculosis.
TCAs. *See* Tricyclic antidepressants.
Teaching, effective
    characteristics of, 21-22
    compliance and, 9-11
    evaluation and, 4-5, 26-27
    and learning, differences between, 4, 5t
    open-ended questions and, 6, 7t
    planning for, 16-21
    special needs and, 21-26, 25t
    traits of, 6-9
Temazepam, 220
Tendinitis and bursitis, 166-167
TENS. *See* Transcutaneous electrical nerve stimulation.
Terazosin, 168
Terbutaline, 58, 60
Tetracaine, 122

Tetracycline, 60, 132, 200
Theophylline, 58
Thiazide diuretics, 40, 44, 46, 141
Thioridazine, 92
Thrombocytopenia, 90-91
Thrombolytic agents, 48
Thrombolytic enzymes, 70
Thymopoietin, 198
Thyroid hormone antagonists, 144
Thyroid hormones, 146
Thyroid replacement drugs, 74
Ticarcillin, 118, 154
Tic douloureux. See Trigeminal neuralgia.
Timolol, 186
Tincture of opium, 218
Tinea. See Dermatophytosis and candidiasis.
Tinnitus, 194-195
Tobramycin, 214
Tocainide, 194
Tolbutamide, 130, 138
Topical anesthetics, 122. See also Anesthetics.
Topical steroids, 122
Tracheobronchitis. See Bronchitis.
Tramadol, 150, 152, 154, 160
Transcutaneous electrical nerve stimulation, 263-264
Transdermal estradiol, 142, 232, 236
Transdermal fentanyl, 226
Trazodone, 92, 152, 216, 220
Triamcinolone, 90, 166, 192, 198, 214
Triazolam, 220
Trichomoniasis. See Vaginitis.
Tricyclic antidepressants, 100, 247
Triethanolamine, 160
Trigeminal neuralgia, 110-111
Trihexyphenidyl, 106
Trimethaphan, 71
Trimethoprim, 182, 183
Trimethoprim-sulfamethoxazole, 172
Troglitazone, 138, 236
Tuberculosis, 76-77

U

Ulcerative colitis. See Inflammatory bowel disease.
Uricosurics, 140
Urinary incontinence, 180-181
Urinary tract infection, 182-183
Ursodiol, 112
UTI. See Urinary tract infection.

V

Vaginitis, 242-243
Valacyclovir, 204
Valproate, 226
Valproic acid, 91, 108
Valvular heart disease, 56-57
Variant angina, 31
Varicella-zoster virus. See Herpes simplex and herpes zoster.
Venlafaxine, 92, 94, 106, 216, 220
Venous stasis ulcers, 214-215
Verapamil, 30, 72
Vertigo, 196-197
Vinblastine, 247
Vincristine, 247
Virchow's triad, 38
Viscous Xylocaine, 190
Vitamin supplements, 64, 72, 86, 108, 112, 114, 124, 148, 162, 178, 208, 220, 224, 232
Vomiting, nausea and cancer and, 222-223
Von Willebrand's disease. See Hemophilia.
VZV. See Herpes simplex and herpes zoster.

WXYZ

Warfarin, 38, 42, 52, 70
Zalcitabine, 82
Zidovudine, 82
Zolpidem, 92, 220